Complete 21-Day Weight Watcher Cookbook :

Flavourful Breakfast, Lunch and Dinner Recipe

By

Sharon S. Lent

Copyright

All rights reserved. No part of the publication maybe reproduced,distributed or transmitted in any form or by any means, including photocopying, recording, or other electronic or mechanical methods, without the prior written permission of the publisher, expect in the case of brief quotation embodied in critical reviews and certain other non-commercial uses permitted by copy right law.

Copyright (Sharon S. Lent),(2024).

Scan me

Get more Access to more helpful books

CONTENT

INTRODUCTION

Breakfast

Lunch

Dinner

Conclusion

ABOUT THE AUTHOR

REVIEW

INTRODUCTION

Embark on a 21-day odyssey of flavors and wellness with Sharon S. Lent, your trusted companion through the pages of the "Complete 21-Day Weight Watch Cookbook." As you open the cover, you're not just entering a realm of recipes but stepping into a world where each dish is a chapter in your transformative journey.

Sharon, a beacon in the realm of nutrition and weight loss, shares her profound insights and culinary prowess to guide you towards a healthier and more vibrant life. This cookbook is not a mere compilation of recipes; it's a testament to her dedication to your well-being.

Picture waking up to the aroma of a perfectly balanced breakfast, where every ingredient is meticulously chosen to kickstart your day with energy and nourishment. Sharon's breakfast recipes are more than just sustenance; they're a celebration of mornings, setting the tone for the day ahead. From hearty oatmeal loaded with fruits to indulgent yet guilt-free smoothies, each breakfast creation is a symphony of flavors designed to make your mornings delightful.

Moving into the heart of the day, Sharon's lunch recipes become your partners in conquering the midday hunger while staying true to your weight loss goals. Bid farewell to bland salads and tasteless wraps as you dive into a world of vibrant salads, wholesome soups, and creatively crafted sandwiches. These lunches are not just meals; they are moments of rejuvenation, ensuring you power through the rest of your day with vitality.

As the sun sets, the dinner table becomes a canvas for Sharon's culinary artistry. Imagine savoring dinners that are not only satisfying to your taste buds but also nurturing to your body. From succulent grilled proteins to inventive vegetable-based dishes, each dinner recipe is a testament to Sharon's commitment to making your weight loss journey flavorful and enjoyable.

What sets this cookbook apart is its holistic approach. Sharon understands that a successful weight loss journey isn't just about what you eat but how you approach food. Throughout the pages, she weaves in insights into mindful eating, portion control, and building a sustainable relationship with food. It's not just a cookbook; it's a guide, a mentor, and a friend, supporting you every step of the way.

The 21-day timeline adds an exciting dimension to this culinary adventure. It's not just about individual meals; it's about the synergy of flavors and nutrients over the course of a month. Each recipe is thoughtfully curated to complement the others, creating a balanced and varied menu that keeps your palate intrigued and your body well-nourished.

In the hustle of daily life, it's easy to succumb to the allure of quick fixes and fad diets. Sharon, however, advocates for a sustainable and enjoyable approach to weight loss. Her cookbook is a testament to the idea that achieving your health goals can be a delightful and enriching experience.

As you turn the pages of the "Complete 21-Day Weight Watcher Cookbook," envision not just the dishes on your plate but the vitality they bring to your life. Sharon S. Lent invites you to savor each moment, appreciate the journey, and discover that a healthier, happier you is within reach one delicious recipe at a time.

Day 1

Breakfast

Scrambled eggs with spinach and feta.

Lunch

Grilled chicken vegetable and avocado salad.

Dinner

Sheet Pan Salmon with Broccoli & Cauliflower.

BREAKFAST

Scrambled eggs with spinach and feta.

INGREDIENTS

4 oz. fresh spinach
4 large eggs
1 Tbsp butter
1 oz. feta
1 pinch crushed red
pepper
1 pinch freshly cracked
black pepper
1 pinch salt

INSTRUCTION

Roughly chop the spinach into smaller pieces (about 1-inch pieces). This step is optional and can be skipped to make breakfast faster, but I prefer the smaller pieces that don't get stringy like whole spinach leaves can tend to be.

Crack the eggs into a large bowl, add a pinch of salt, and whisk (I prefer ribbons of white and yellow, but you can whisk until even if preferred).

Add the butter to a large skillet and melt over medium heat. Add the chopped spinach and sauté until the spinach has softened (2-3 minutes)

Push the sautéed spinach to the outside edges of the skillet and pour the eggs into the center. Gently fold the eggs as the bottom layer solidifies, until the eggs are about 75% solid. Fold the eggs into the sautéed spinach, then turn off the heat. The residual heat in the pan will finish cooking the eggs without overcooking or drying them out.

Top the eggs with the crumbled feta, a little freshly cracked pepper, and a pinch of crushed red pepper, then serve.

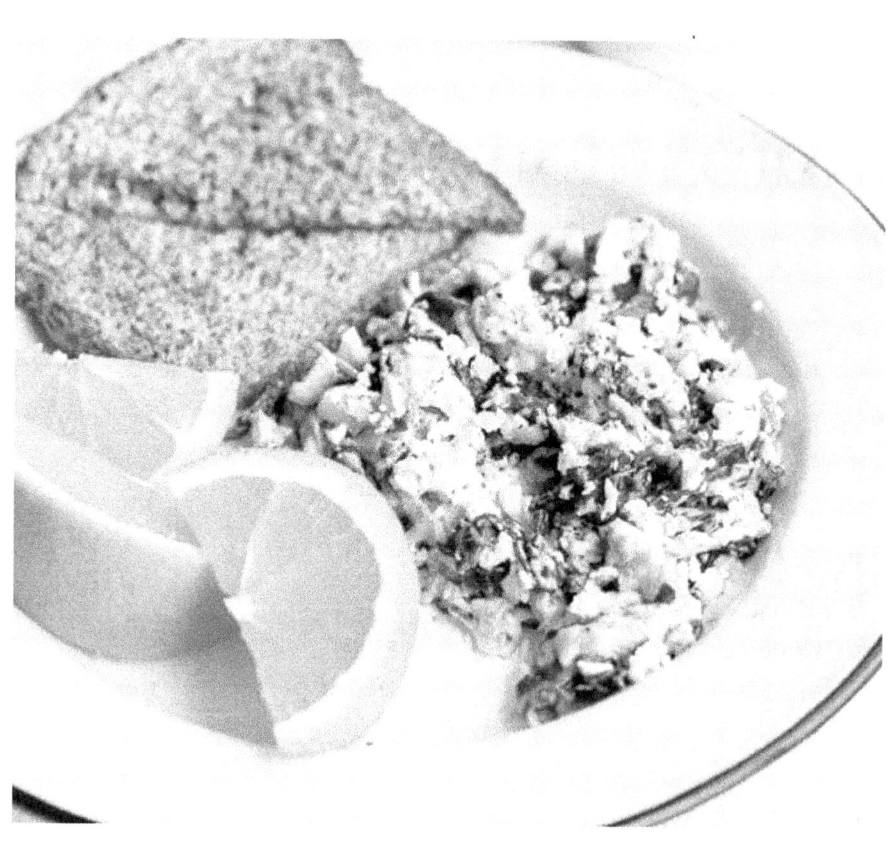

LUNCH

Grilled chicken vegetable and avocado salad.

INGREDIENT

Chicken Marinade:
1/4 cup olive oil
juice of 1 lemon
3 tablespoons low sodium soy sauce
1 tablespoon worcestershire sauce
1/4 cup coconut or brown sugar
1/2 teaspoon garlic powder
1/2 teaspoon onion powder
1 teaspoon kosher salt
pepper, to taste
2 pounds chicken breasts or thighs, boneless and skinless
Vegetables to Grill:
1 eggplant, cut into rounds
2 zucchini, cut lengthwise into flats
1 red onion, cut into wedges
2 ears corn on the cob, shucked
2 avocados, halved and pitted
2 tablespoons olive oil
2 teaspoons kosher salt
Remainder of Salad Ingredients:
1 cup cherry tomatoes, halved (or 1 whole tomato cut into
wedges)
2 heads romaine or baby gem lettuce
1 recipe Citrus Herb Vinaigrette or favorite store bought
vinaigrette

INSTRUCTION

Place the ¼ cup olive oil, lemon juice, soy sauce, Worcestershire sauce, sugar, garlic powder, onion powder, 1 tsp of salt and pepper in a bowl or bag and whisk to combine.

Add chicken to the marinade for at least 30 minutes on the counter and up to 5 hours refrigerated.

Place the vegetables in a bowl or on a baking sheet, brush with 2 tbsp olive oil and sprinkle with 2 tsp salt making sure all surfaces are coated.

Preheat grill to medium/high heat.

Place the chicken on the grill and cook for 6-7 minutes per side or until chicken is firm to the touch and golden or until a meat thermometer reads 160°F.

Grill the vegetables for several minutes per side or until golden and fork tender.

Remove the chicken and vegetables to a large plate or baking sheet and cool.

Place the lettuce and tomatoes on a large wooden board or salad platter.

Chop the chicken and vegetables into desired sized pieces leaving the avocado halves whole to scoop out and place on top of each salad.

Top greens with grilled chicken, vegetables and tomatoes.

Drizzle with Citrus Herb Vinaigrette or favorite store bought vinaigrette.

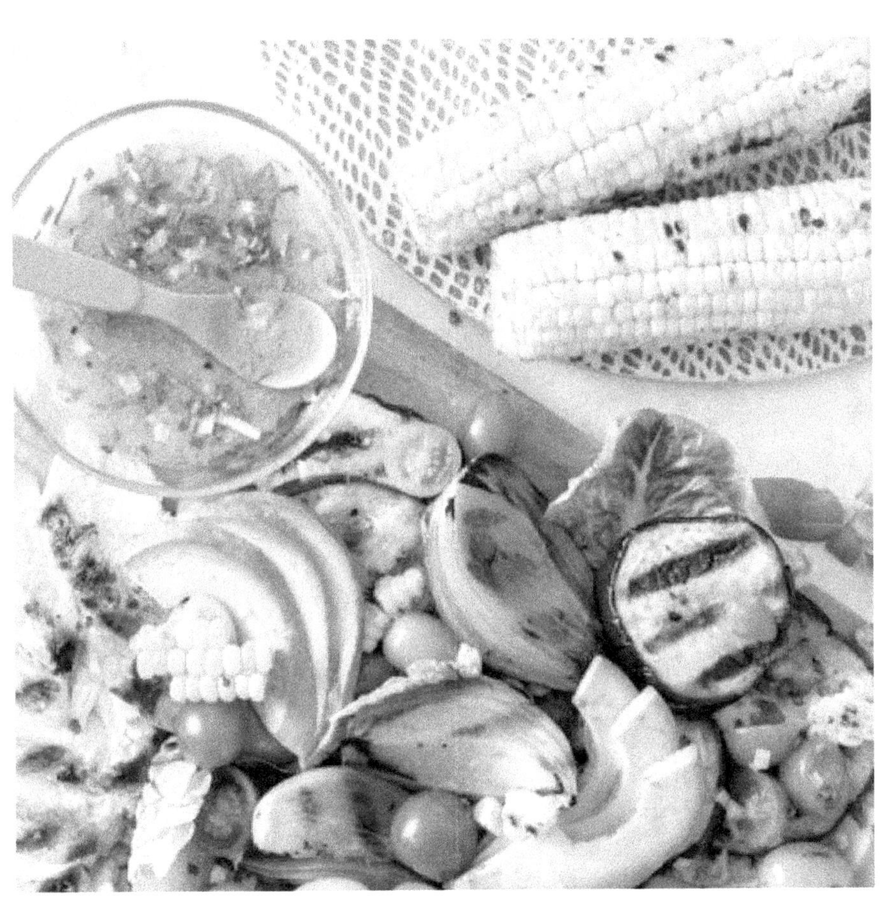

DINNER
Sheet Pan Salmon with Broccoli & Cauliflower

INGREDIENT

1 tbsp
olive oi
1
lemon, juic
1/2 tsp
garlic powde
1/2 tsp
red pepper flake
2 cups
broccoli floret
2 cups
cauliflower floret
4
salmon fillets (4oz
Salt and pepper to taste

INSTRUCTION

Preheat the oven to 400°F.

Arrange broccoli and cauliflower florets on a sheet pan. Season with olive oil, garlic, red pepper flakes, lemon juice, salt and pepper. Bake for 8 to 10 minutes.

Remove sheet pan from oven and arrange salmon fillets in the centre of the pan. Season the salmon with olive oil, garlic, red pepper flakes, lemon juice, salt and pepper. Bake for an additional 10 to 15 minutes or until salmon is cooked to your liking.

Serve immediately or store in the refrigerator for up to 3 days.

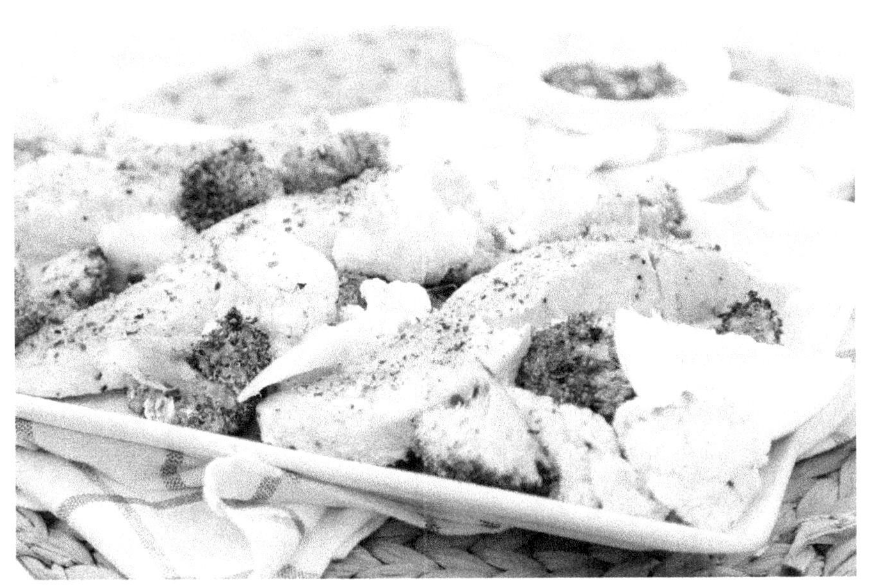

Day 2

Breakfast

Greek yogurt parfait with berries and almonds.

Lunch

Turkey lettuce wraps.

Dinner

Zucchini noodles with pesto and grilled chicken.

BREAKFAST

Greek yogurt parfait with berries and almonds.

INGREDIENTS

4 each strawberries, fresh
quartered
½ cup blueberries, fresh
½ cup plain Greek yogurt
1 tsp almonds, toasted (a total
of ½ cup for toasting and use
at a later time)
1 tsp honey

INSTRUCTION

Place ½ cup almonds in a cast-iron skillet over medium-high heat.
Stir with a spoon until they turn a light brown. Watch them
carefully because once they start browning they can burn easily.
Remove from heat and let cool.

I like to store the extra almonds in a small mason jar.
Roasted Almonds in a small glass jar
ASSEMBLE YOGURT PARFAIT
Rinse strawberries under running water. Remove green stems.
Strawberries in a wire strainer
Quarter strawberries and place in a serving bowl.
Strawberries in a glass bowl and a white round bowl
Rinse blueberries under running water. Remove stems.
Blueberries in a wire strainer
Place blueberries on top of the strawberries.
Blueberries on top of strawberries in a glass bowl and white bowl
Measure yogurt and spoon on top of the blueberries.
Yogurt on top of berries in a glass bowl and a white bowl
Sprinkle almonds on top of the yogurt.
Yogurt and Berry Parfait
Drizzle parfaits with honey.
Yogurt and Berries topped with roasted almonds in a white bowl
and glass bowl8.   Enjoy!

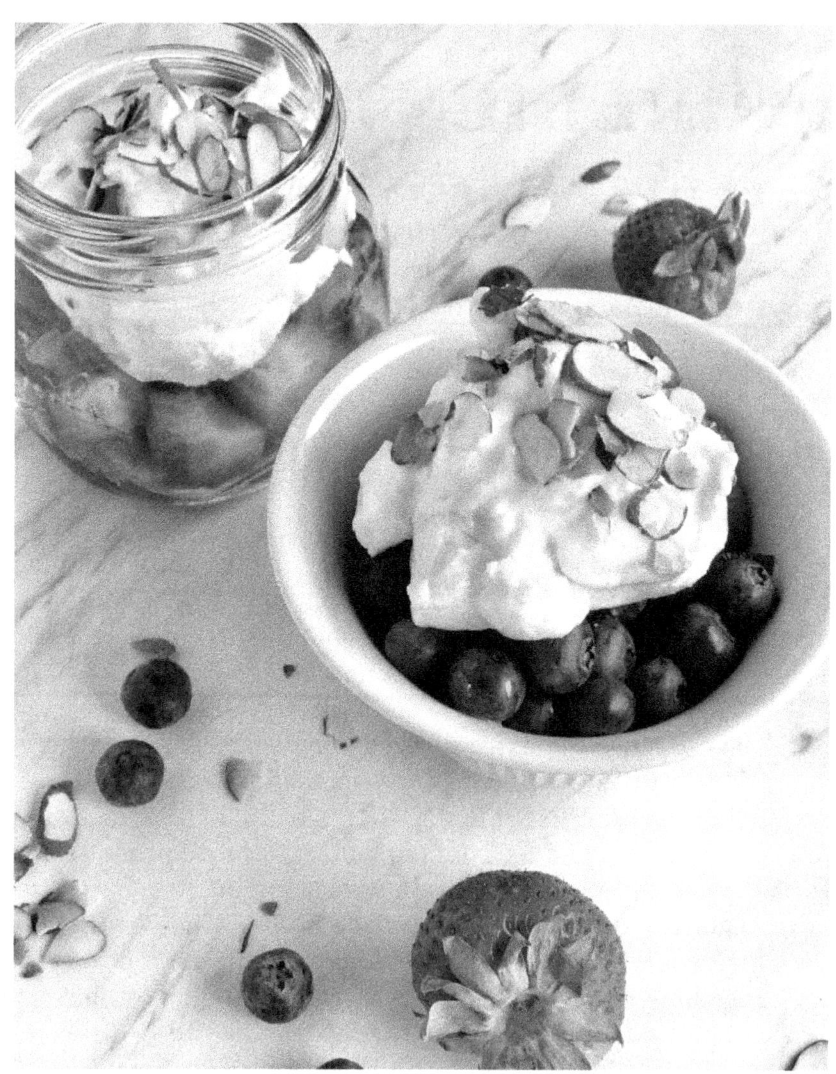

LUNCH
Turkey lettuce wraps

INGREDIENT

Mission Gluten-Free Tortillas
Romaine Lettuce leaves
Turkey sliced
Cheese sliced
avocado sliced
Cucumber thinly sliced lengthwise
Italian Salad Dressing

INSTRUCTION

Layer lettuce, turkey, cheese, avocado, and cucumber in tortilla and roll up tight, placing with the edges down to keep from unraveling.

Pack salad dressing in a cup on the side for dipping.

Include some berries and a treat of graham crackers to complete this simple, nutritious meal!

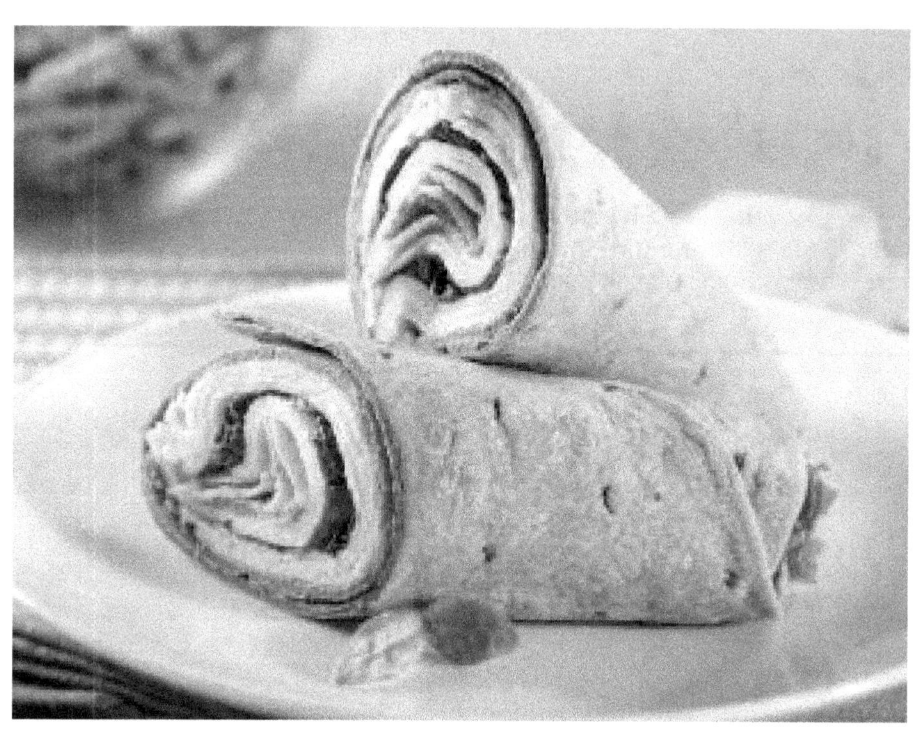

DINNER

Zucchini noodles with pesto and grilled chicken.

INGREDIENTS

4 medium-large zucchini (about 2 pounds), trimmed

¾ teaspoon salt, divided

2 cups packed fresh basil leaves

¼ cup pine nuts, toasted

¼ cup grated Parmesan cheese

1/4 cup plus 2 tablespoons extra-virgin olive oil, divided

2 tablespoons lemon juice

1 large clove garlic, quartered

½ teaspoon ground pepper

1 pound boneless, skinless chicken breast, cut into 1-inch pieces

INSTRUCTION

Using a spiral vegetable slicer, cut zucchini lengthwise into long, thin strands. Give the strands a chop here and there so the noodles aren't too long. Place the zucchini in a colander and toss with 1/4 teaspoon salt. Let drain for 15 to 30 minutes, then gently squeeze to remove any excess liquid.

Meanwhile, place basil, pine nuts, Parmesan, 1/4 cup oil, lemon juice, garlic, pepper and 1/4 teaspoon salt in a mini food processor. Process until almost smooth.

Heat 1 tablespoon oil in a large skillet over medium-high heat. Add chicken in one layer; sprinkle with the remaining 1/4 teaspoon salt. Cook, stirring, until just cooked through, about 5 minutes. Transfer to a large bowl and stir in 3 tablespoons of the pesto.

Add the remaining 1 tablespoon oil to the pan. Add the drained zucchini noodles and toss gently until hot, 2 to 3 minutes. Transfer to the bowl with the chicken. Add the remaining pesto and toss gently to coat.

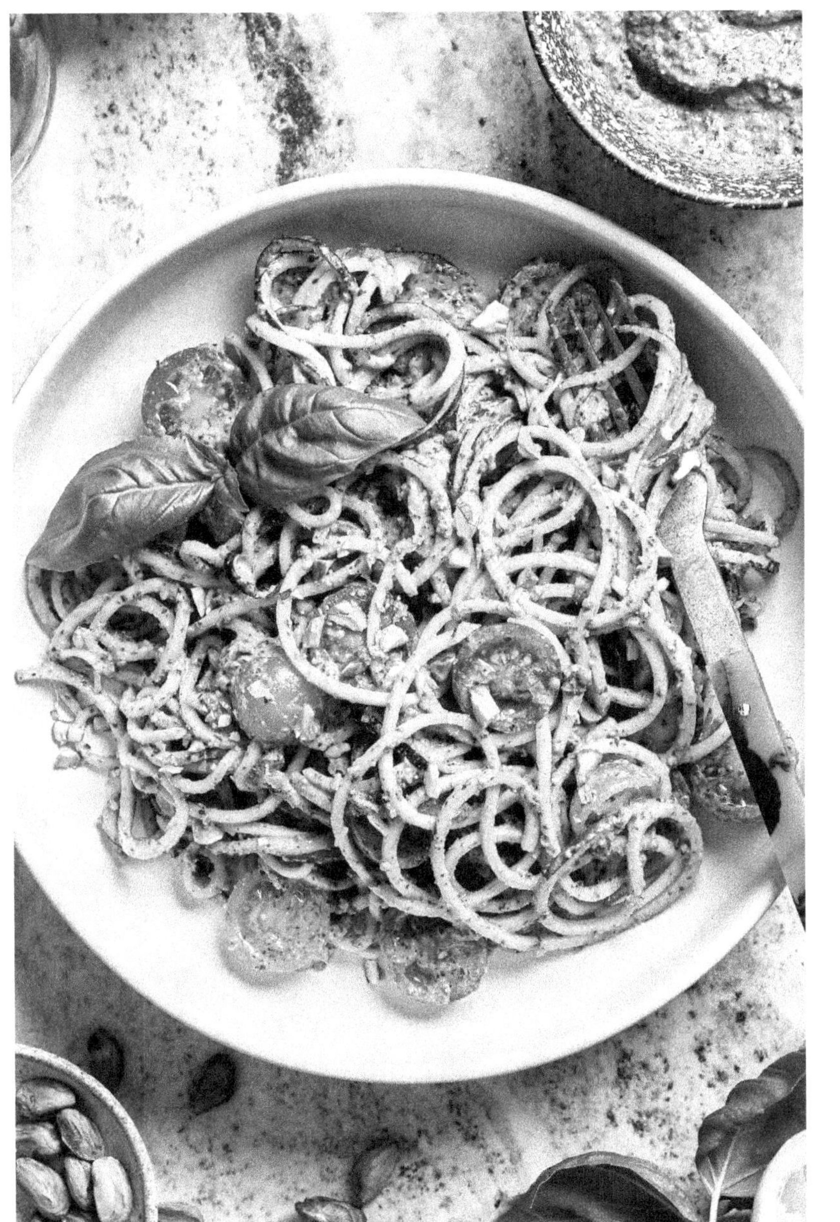

Day 3

Breakfast

Omelette with mushrooms, onions, and cheese.

Lunch

Quinoa salad with grilled vegetables and chickpeas.

Dinner

Beef and vegetable stir-fry.

Breakfast

Omelette with mushrooms, onions, and cheese.

INGREDIENTS

1 tablespoon Hiland Butter
1/2 Onion, medium, finely chopped
125 grams Fresh Mushrooms, washed
and thinly sliced
Salt and Freshly Ground Pepper, to
taste
3 Eggs, large, lightly beaten
1-2 tablespoons Shredded Hiland Mild
Cheddar cheese (optional)

INSTRUCTION

Melt Hiland Butter over medium heat in a 9 or 10 inch skillet. Add onions and saute for 2-3 minutes. Add mushrooms and saute until soft. Remove onions and mushrooms and place in bowl.

Wipe skillet clean with a paper towel. Spray well with non-stick spray.

Pour lightly beaten eggs into skillet so that the whole skillet is covered. Cover the skillet. Cook on low flame.

After a minute or two, when egg begins to set, gently lift the edges of the egg with a spatula so that the uncooked egg in the middle runs to the edges of the pan and cooks. Cover again. If needed, repeat the process of running uncooked egg out of the middle of the omelet.

When the egg has started to set, place the onions and mushrooms on half of the eggs. Sprinkle the Hiland Cheddar Cheese on top of the onions and mushrooms. Carefully fold the other half of the omelet over the filling. Cover. Cook on low for another minute or two, just until the cheese is melted.

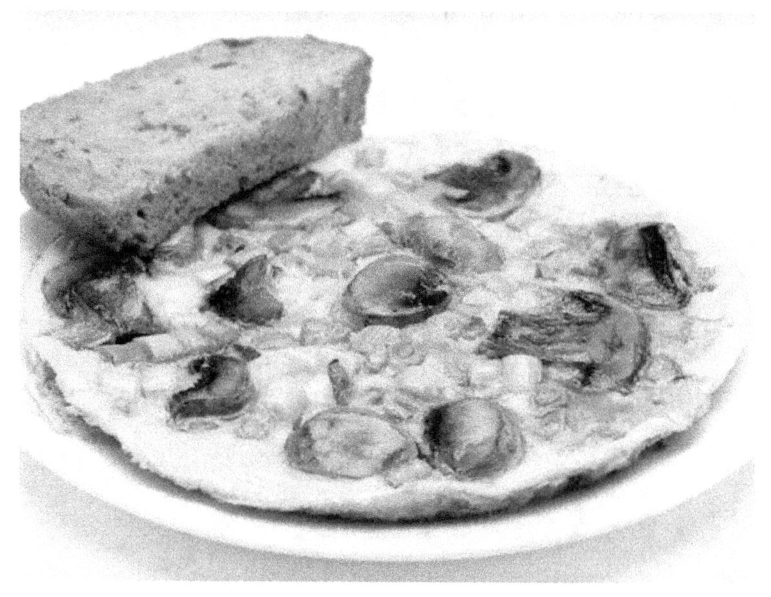

LUNCH

Quinoa salad with grilled vegetables and chickpeas.

INGREDIENTS

2 red or yellow peppers, deseeded and cut into chunks
1 red onion, cut into small wedges
2 large beetroot, peeled and cut into small wedges
4 garlic cloves, unpeeled
4 tbsp olive oil
200g quinoa
480ml vegetable stock (check it's vegan and gluten free)
400g tin chickpeas, drained and rinsed
1 ripe avocado, stoned, peeled and sliced
For the citrus dressing

Juice 1 lemon
2 tsp sumac
Pinch caster sugar
A few fresh coriander or flatleaf parsley sprigs, chopped

INSTRUCTION

Heat the oven to 200°C/180°C fan/ gas 6. Put the peppers, onion and beetroot in a roasting tin, tuck the garlic cloves in between, then drizzle with the olive oil to coat everything. Roast for 25-30 minutes or until tender. Squeeze the garlic cloves out of their skins and mix the flesh into the vegetables (discard the skins). Meanwhile, rinse the quinoa under cold running water and drain in a sieve. Bring the stock to the boil in a saucepan, add the quinoa and reduce the heat to a simmer. Cover and cook for 15 minutes until the quinoa is tender and has absorbed most of the stock. When cooked, the sprout or 'tail' will pop out of each quinoa seed. Remove from the heat and leave for 5 minutes before straining off any excess stock. Fluff up the quinoa with a fork. Mix together the quinoa, roasted vegetables (reserving the oil left in the roasting tin), chickpeas and avocado in a serving bowl. Whisk the dressing ingredients with the reserved oil from the roasting tin and gently toss with the salad. Serve warm.

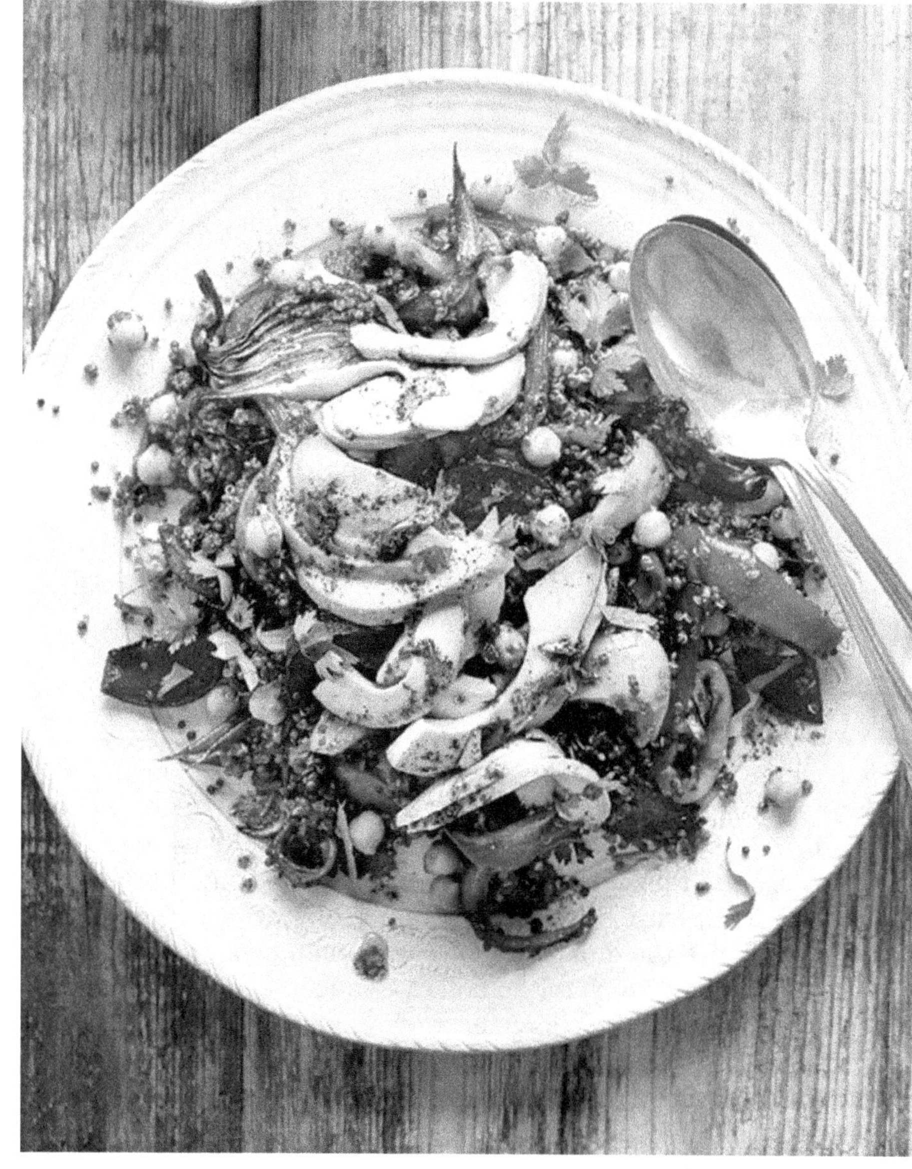

DINNER

Beef and vegetable stir-fry.

INGREDIENTS

12 ounces top sirloin, trimmed of excess fat & thinly sliced against the grain (see Recipe Notes)
1 tablespoon cornstarch
1 tablespoon soy sauce
1 tablespoon Shaoxing wine (see Recipe Notes)
1/4 teaspoon white pepper
stir fry vegetables (see Recipe Notes)
1/2 small head broccoli, cut into small bite-sized florets (~3.5 oz or ~1 cup florets)
1 large carrot, peeled as desired & sliced into 1/8-inch thick strips (~3.5 oz or ~1 cup sliced)
1 small red onion, thinly sliced (~3.5 oz or ~1.5 cups sliced)
1/2 large red bell pepper, chopped into 1-inch pieces (~3.5 oz or ~1 cup sliced)
3-4 mushrooms (white button or cremini/baby bella), trimmed & thinly sliced (~4 oz or ~2 cups sliced)
1/2 small napa cabbage, chopped into 1-inch pieces (~4.5 oz or ~2 cups chopped)
large handful snow peas, ends trimmed as desired (~2.5 oz or ~3/4 cup)
4 teaspoons grapeseed oil or high smoke point vegetable oil of choice
kosher salt & white pepper, to season
for serving, as desired: cooked white rice or grain of choice, thinly sliced green onions, toasted sesame seeds, etc.
for the stir fry sauce:

3/4 cup beef stock
1 tablespoon cornstarch
1 tablespoon dark brown sugar (can sub regular brown sugar)
2 tablespoons oyster sauce
1 tablespoon soy sauce
2 teaspoons sesame oil, divided
2 cloves garlic, finely chopped or grated

INSTRUCTION

Marinate the beef: Add thinly sliced top sirloin, cornstarch, soy sauce, & rice wine to a medium bowl. Season with white pepper. Stir to combine, coating the beef thoroughly & evenly. Set aside to rest at room temperature while you prepare the rest of the ingredients. This is a great time to prepare all of the stir fry vegetables, chopping & slicing everything as indicated in the Ingredients List, above.

Prepare the stir fry sauce: Add the beef stock cornstarch, dark brown sugar, oyster sauce, soy sauce, & 1 teaspoon of the sesame oil to a small bowl or jar. Whisk or shake to combine well. Set aside. Add the remaining 1 teaspoon sesame oil to a small saucepan over medium-high heat. Once hot, add the garlic & cook until fragrant & lightly browned, 30 seconds – 1 minute. Stir in the beef stock mixture & cook, stirring occasionally, until thickened, 4-5 minutes. Remove from the heat & set aside.

Stir fry the vegetables: Meanwhile, as the stir fry sauce thickens, begin the stir fry. Add 1 teaspoon of the grapeseed oil to a wok or large skillet over medium-high heat. Once hot & shimmering, add the carrots & broccoli. Lightly season with a small pinch of salt & cook, stirring often, until vibrantly colored & softened slightly, 3-4 minutes. Transfer to a large plate or bowl & set aside. Add another 1 teaspoon of oil to the wok or skillet & return to medium-high heat. Once hot & shimmering, add the sliced red onion, bell pepper, mushrooms, cabbage, & snow peas. Lightly season with a small pinch of salt & cook, stirring often, until softened slightly, about 3 minutes. Transfer to the same large plate or bowl as the broccoli & carrots & set aside.

Sear the beef & finish the stir fry: Add the remaining 2 teaspoon of oil to the wok or skillet & reduce the heat to medium. Once hot & shimmering, add the marinated beef from Step 1. Shake the pan to separate the slices of beef for even browning. Cook, tossing & stirring occasionally, just until browned. While stirring, pour the prepared stir fry sauce from Step 2 into the skillet. Add the stir fried vegetables back into the skillet. Cook 1-2 minutes longer, tossing & stirring frequently to bring the beef and vegetable stir fry together. Remove from the heat.

Serve immediately, spooning the beef and vegetable stir fry over rice or grain of choice. Finish with thinly sliced green onions & toasted sesame seeds as desired. Enjoy!Serve immediately, spooning the beef and vegetable stir fry over rice or grain of choice. Finish with thinly sliced green onions & toasted sesame seeds as desired. Enjoy!

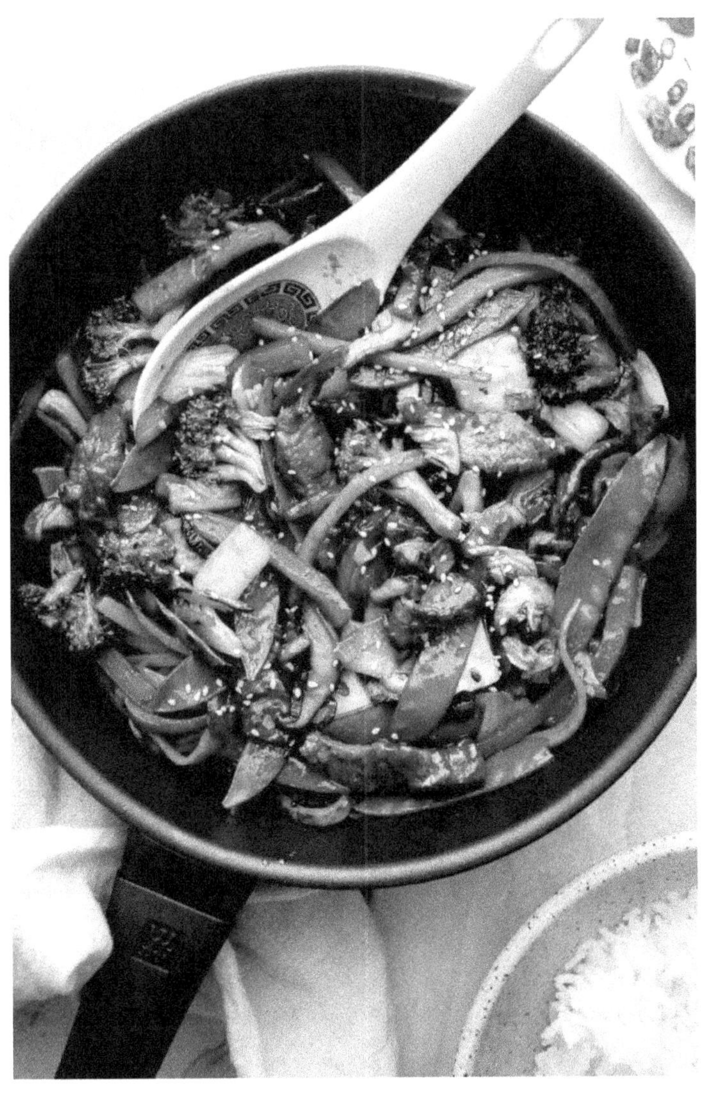

Day 4

Breakfast

Avocado and smoked salmon on whole grain toast.

Lunch

Zucchini noodles with shrimp and garlic.

Dinner

Cauliflower crust pizza with assorted veggies .

Breakfast

Avocado and smoked salmon on whole grain toast.

INGREDIENTS

2 pieces toast multi-grain bread and sourdough bread
would all work
1 large avocado ripene
1 ½ teaspoons lemon juice plus lemon wedges to serve
wit
1 garlic clove minced – optiona
½ teaspoon Kosher sal
¼ teaspoon ground black peppe
½ Persian cucumber peeled and sliced thinly (or
English cucumber would also work
4 oz. smoked salmon package
½ cup micro greens or arugul
1 tablespoon pickled red onions optiona
A drizzle of extra virgin olive oi
1 teaspoon Everything Bagel Seasoning optiona
lllad)rtlhdg optional

INSTRUCTION

If preferred, toast your bread and let it cool for
a few minutes.
Meanwhile, in a small bowl, mash avocado using
the back of a fork. Add lemon juice, minced
garlic (if using), salt, and pepper. Stir well. Give
it a taste and add more if necessary.
Spread each slice of toast with the avocado
mixture.
Top each slice with the cucumber slices.
Place smoked salmon pieces and pickled onion
(if using) on top.
Garnish with microgreens and a drizzle of olive
oil. Finish it off with a sprinkle of Everything
Bagel Seasoning.
Serve with a lemon wedge on the side.

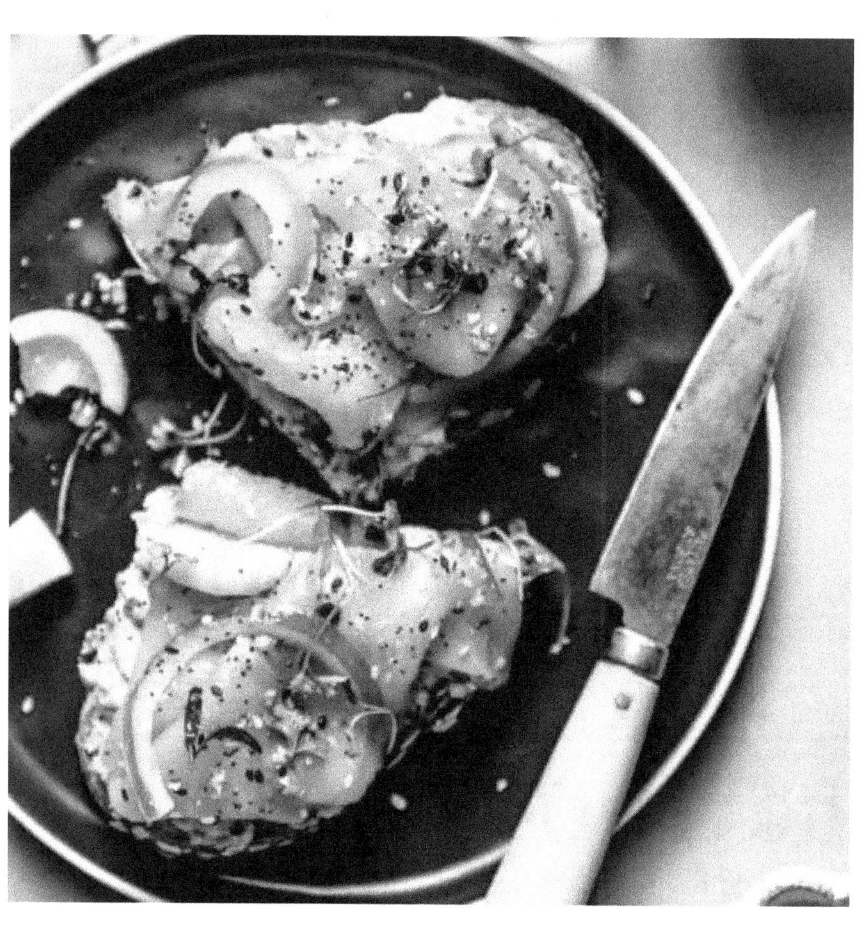

LUNCH

Zucchini noodles with shrimp and garlic.

INGREDIENTS

4 tablespoons unsalted butter, divided
4 cloves garlic, minced and divided
1 pound 3 medium-sized zucchini,
spiralized*
Kosher salt and freshly ground black
pepper, to taste
1 shallot, minced
1 pound medium shrimp, peeled and
deveined
2 teaspoons lemon zest
2 tablespoons chopped fresh parsley leaves

INSTRUCTION

Melt 1 tablespoon butter in a large skillet over medium heat. Add 2 cloves garlic and cook, stirring frequently, until fragrant, about 1 minute.
Stir in zucchini noodles until just tender, about 2-3 minutes; season with salt and pepper, to taste. Set aside and keep warm.
Melt the remaining 3 tablespoons butter in the skillet. Add remaining 2 cloves garlic and shallot, and cook, stirring frequently, until fragrant, about 2 minutes.
Add shrimp; season with salt and pepper, to taste. Cook, stirring occasionally, until pink and cooked through, about 3-4 minutes. Stir in lemon zest and parsley.
Serve immediately with zucchini noodles.

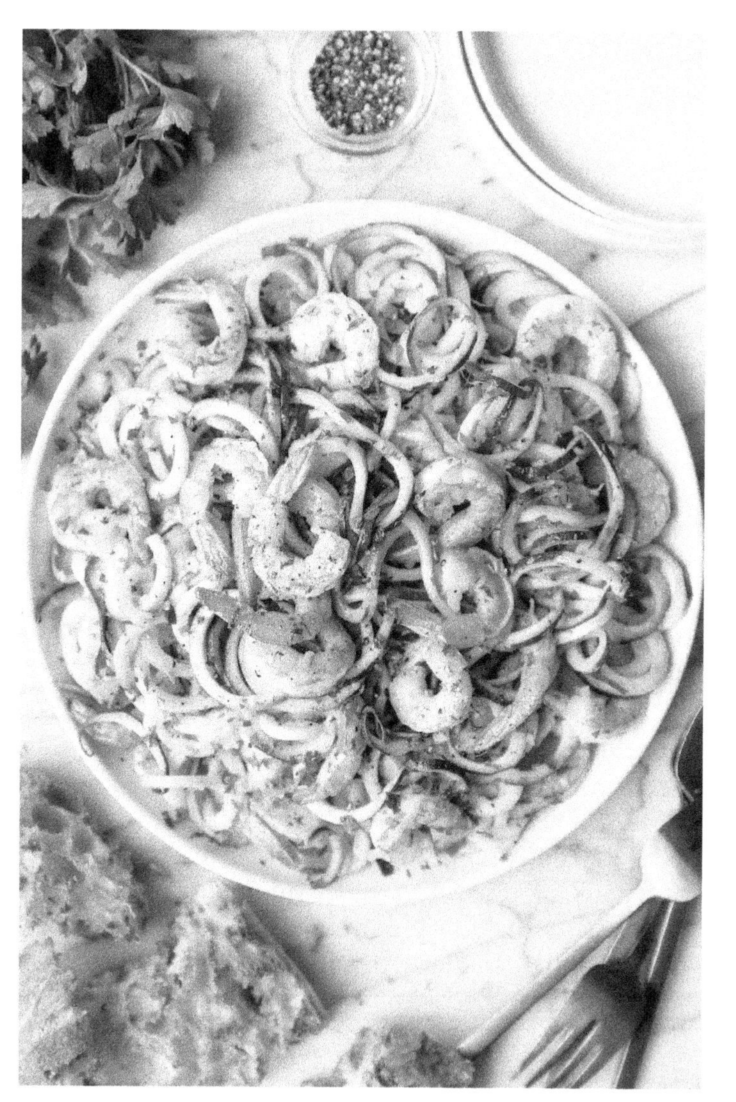

DINNER

Cauliflower crust pizza with assorted veggies

INGREDIENTS

1 cauliflower head, roughly chopped (about 3 pound
Cooking spr
2 teaspoons olive oil, divid
½ cup presliced cremini mushroo
½ cup sliced red bell pepp
½ cup thinly sliced fresh basil, divid
¼ teaspoon freshly ground black pepper, divid
⅛ teaspoon kosher sa
3 garlic cloves, minc
2 ½ ounces shredded part-skim mozzarella cheese
(about 2/3 cup), divid
2 large egg whit
½ ounces grated Parmesan chee
½ cup thinly sliced seeded tomato
⅔ cup fresh baby
spinachesseesededltededermsedays)tsTo):r:s:yR
yretn5re ss ttses thinly sliced seeded tomatoes
⅔ cup fresh baby spinach

INSTRUCTION

Step 1
Preheat oven to 375°.

ADVERTISEMENT

Step 2
Place half of cauliflower in a food processor; pulse 10 to 15 times or until finely chopped (like rice). Transfer cauliflower to a baking sheet lined with parchment paper. Repeat procedure with remaining cauliflower. Coat cauliflower with cooking spray. Bake at 375° for 25 minutes, stirring once. Cool.

Step 3
Increase oven temp to 450°.

Step 4
Heat a large skillet over medium-high heat. Add 1 teaspoon oil to pan; swirl to coat. Add mushrooms and bell pepper; sauté 5 minutes or until tender. Set aside.

Step 5
Place cauliflower in a clean kitchen towel. Squeeze until very dry. Combine cauliflower, remaining 1 teaspoon oil, 1/4 cup basil, 1/8 teaspoon black pepper, salt, garlic, 2 ounces mozzarella cheese, egg whites, and Parmesan cheese in a bowl. Press cauliflower mixture into 2 (8-inch) circles on a baking sheet lined with parchment paper. Coat crusts with cooking spray.

Step 6
Bake crusts at 450° for 22 minutes or until browned. Remove pan from oven; top crusts evenly with mushroom mixture, tomatoes, spinach, remaining 1/4 cup basil, remaining 1/8 teaspoon black pepper, and remaining mozzarella cheese. Bake an additional 7 minutes or until cheese melts.

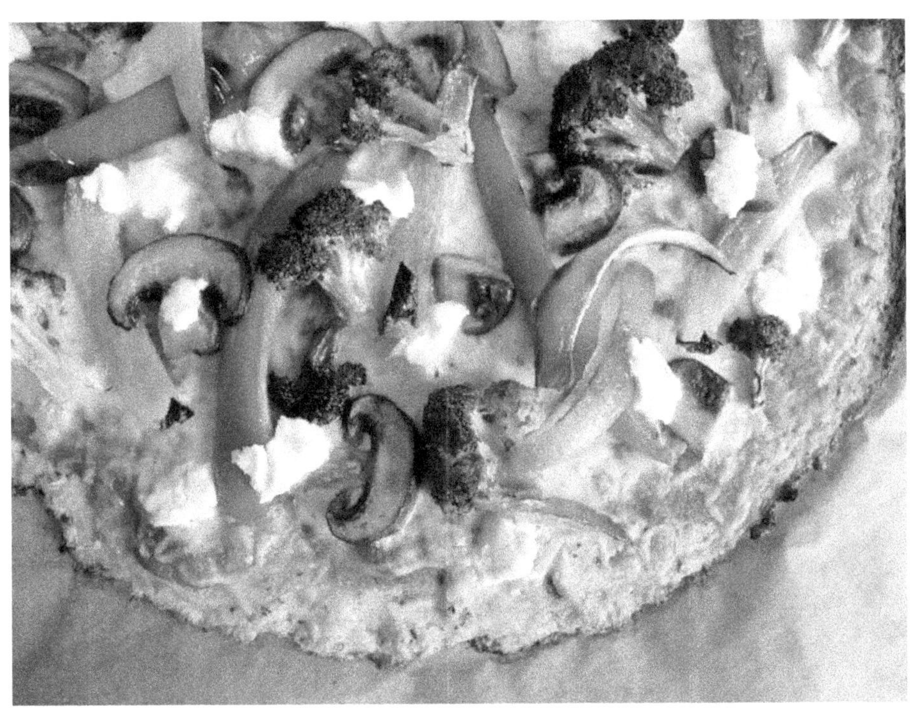

Day 5

Breakfast

Chia seed pudding with unsweetened almond milk.

Lunch

Cobb salad with bacon, eggs, and blue cheese.

Dinner

Grilled shrimp skewers with a side of roasted Brussels sprouts.

BREAKFAST

Chia seed pudding with unsweetened almond milk.

INGREDIENTS

2 tbsp chia seeds

½ cup unsweetened almond milk

1 tbsp honey or other sweetener or to taste

INSTRUCTION

To a small bowl or measuring cup add the almond milk
and honey and mix well.
Whisk in the chia seeds
Refrigerate for 30 minutes and then whisk again
Cover and refrigerate for 4-5 hours, or overnight until
thickened
Stir well before serving.
Add your favorite toppings and serve.

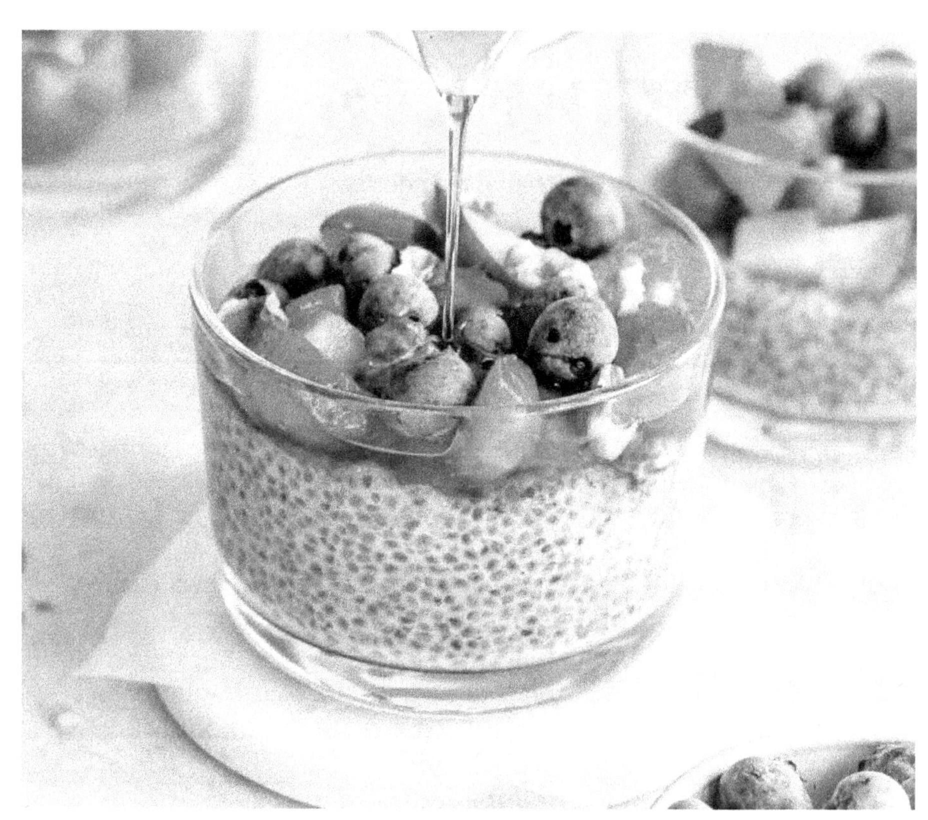

LUNCH

Cobb salad with bacon, eggs, and blue cheese.

INGREDIENTS

6 slices bacon

3 eggs

1 head iceberg lettuce, shredded

3 cups chopped, cooked chicken meat

2 tomatoes, seeded and chopped

¾ cup blue cheese, crumbled

3 green onions, chopped

1 avocado - peeled, pitted and diced

1 (8 ounce) bottle Ranch-style salad dressing

INSTRUCTION

Place eggs in a saucepan and cover completely with cold water; bring to a boil, then cover and remove from heat. Let eggs sit for 10 to 12 minutes, then cool, peel and chop.

While the eggs are cooking, place bacon in a large, deep skillet. Cook over medium-high heat until evenly brown, 7 to 10 minutes. Drain, crumble, and set aside.

Divide shredded lettuce among individual plates. Top with rows of bacon, eggs, chicken, tomatoes, blue cheese, green onions, and avocado.

Drizzle with dressing.

Enjoy ●

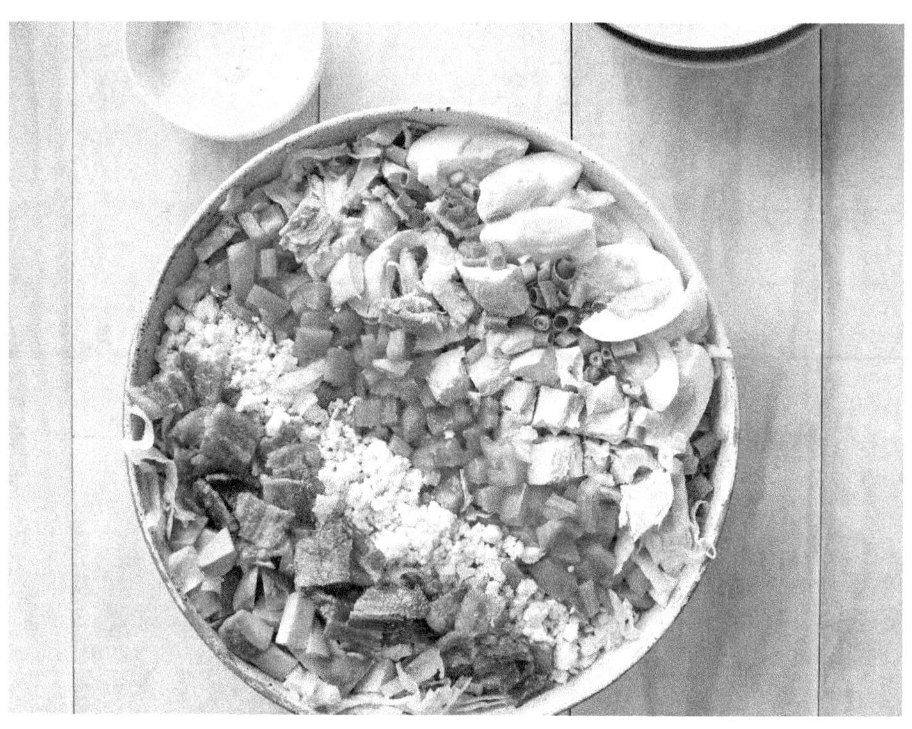

DINNER

Grilled shrimp skewers with a side of roasted Brussels sprouts.

INGREDIENTS

1 pound shrimp, peeled and deveined
3 cloves garlic, minced
2 tbsp fresh lemon juice
2 tbsp olive oil
Salt and black pepper to taste
fresh parsley, for garnish

INSTRUCTION

Preheat your grill to medium-high heat.
In a bowl, combine the minced garlic, lemon juice, olive oil, salt, and black pepper. Mix well.

Add the shrimp to the bowl and toss until they are evenly coated with the marinade. Let it marinate for about 10 minutes.

Thread the shrimp onto skewers, making sure to leave a little space between each shrimp.

Place the shrimp skewers on the preheated grill and cook for about 2-3 minutes per side, or until they turn pink and opaque. Be careful not to overcook them, as they can become rubbery.

Once cooked, remove the shrimp skewers from the grill and transfer them to a serving platter.

Garnish with freshly chopped parsley and squeeze some additional lemon juice over the top, if desired.

Serve hot and enjoy!

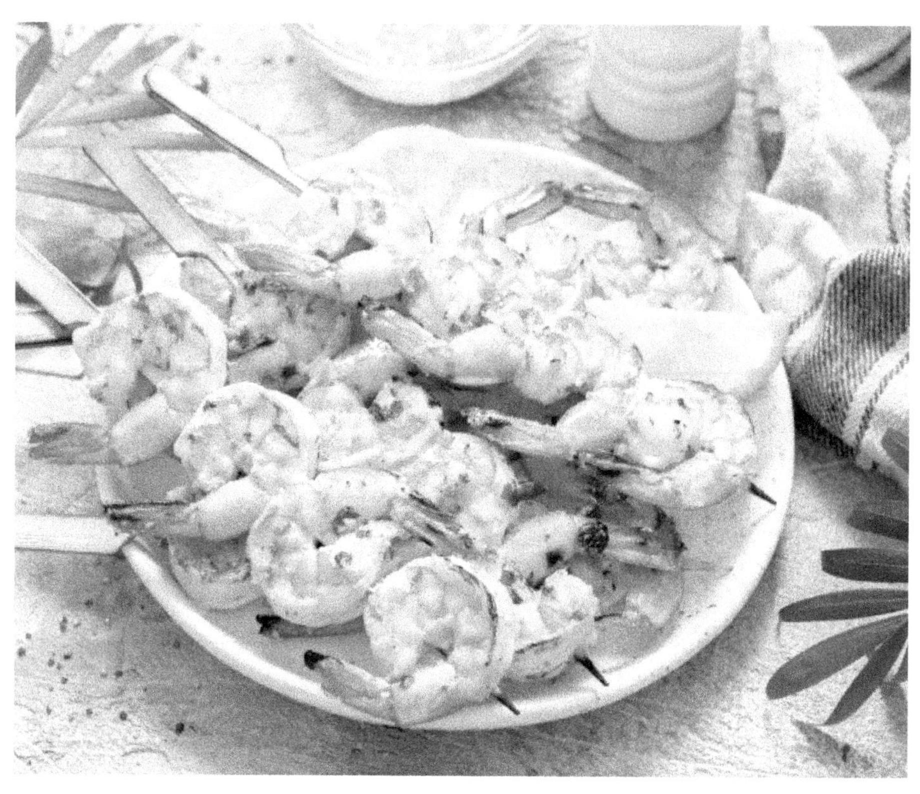

Day 6

Breakfast

Spinach and feta-stuffed chicken breast.

Lunch

Cottage cheese and cherry tomatoes with a sprinkle of chives.

Dinner

Chicken thighs with lemon and rosemary, served with asparagus.

BREAKFAST

Spinach and feta-stuffed chicken breast.

INGREDIENTS

1 tablespoon olive oil

1 cup chopped yellow onion

2 tablespoons chopped fresh dill

5 ounces baby spinach

2 ounces crumbled feta cheese (about 1/2 cup)

4 (6 ounce) skinless, boneless chicken breasts

½ teaspoon kosher salt

¼ teaspoon black pepper

1 ½ teaspoons olive oil

INSTRUCTION

Heat a large skillet over medium heat. Add 1 tablespoon olive oil to pan. Add onion; cook 8 minutes, stirring frequently. Remove pan from heat; stir in dill, spinach and feta cheese. Cool 10 minutes. Cut a horizontal slit through the center of each chicken breast to form a pocket. Stuff each pocket evenly with spinach mixture. Close pockets with toothpicks. Sprinkle with salt and pepper. Heat skillet over medium-high heat. Add 1 1/2 teaspoons olive oil to pan. Add chicken; cook 4 minutes. Turn chicken. Cover pan, reduce heat to medium and cook 5 minutes or until chicken is done.

Serve and enjoy ●

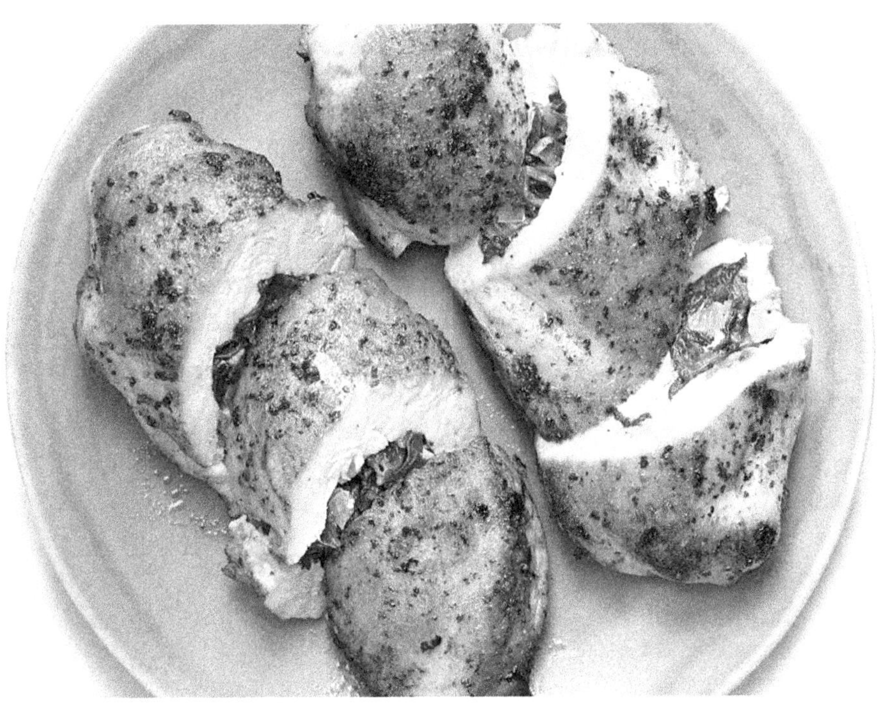

LUNCH

Cottage cheese and cherry tomatoes with a sprinkle of chives.

INGREDIENTS

1/4 teaspoon garlic powder
1/4 teaspoon onion powder
1/4 teaspoon salt
1 1/2 teaspoon chopped fresh chives
2 cups Daisy Brand Low Fat Cottage Cheese
32 cherry tomatoes

INSTRUCTION

Place cottage cheese in a strainer to drain extra liquid. Put cottage cheese, garlic powder, onion powder, salt and chopped chives in a food processor. Blend until smooth.

Pour mixture in a zip-top bag and place in the refrigerator.

Slice the tops off the cherry tomatoes (if desired presentation is to stand stand up, remove a small slice off the bottom to make flat).

Use a small paring knife to core out centers of tomatoes. Cut a small hole in the corner of the zip-top bag. Pip the cottage cheese mixture to fill the centers of the tomatoes.

Reuse the bottoms of cherry tomatoes to place on top and a sprig of parsley for decoration.

Serve immediately. Refrigerate left-overs.

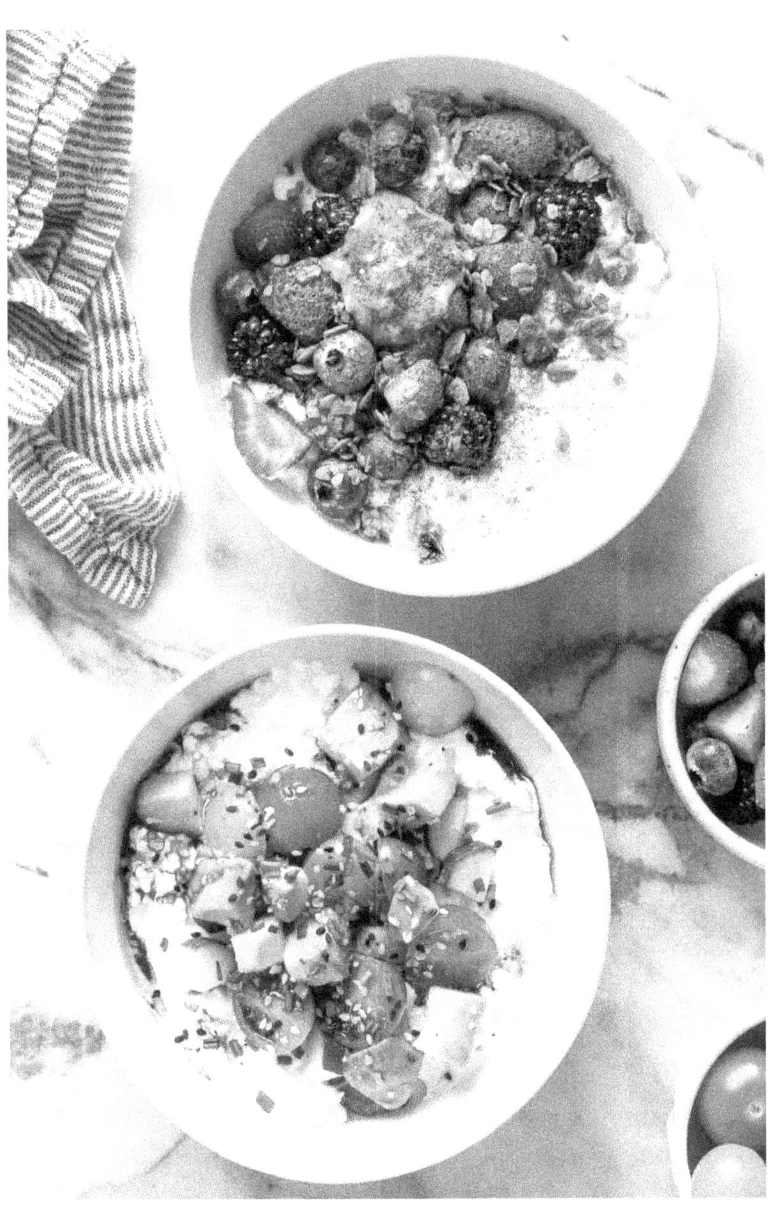

DINNER

Chicken thighs with lemon and rosemary, served with asparagus.

INGREDIENTS

1/2 cup olive oil I used lemon flavoured for a
SUPER lemon boost!
1/4 cup lemon juice
2 tablespoons minced fresh garlic
2 tablespoons dried rosemary or 1/3 cup fresh
1 teaspoon sea salt
3-4 chicken breasts
1 pound of fresh asparagus washed and
trimmed
Extra sea salt and pepper for serving

INSTRUCTION

Combine the first five ingredients in a food processor - or in a container that you can use a hand blender in- and process until creamy and smooth.

Place the chicken in a container and using 1/3 of the sauce, baste. Cover the chicken and the remaining sauce and refrigerate for a few hours.

To cook, preheat your oven to 350 °F.

Remove the chicken from the fridge and place on a large baking sheet or large pan.

Bake for 20 minutes, then add the asparagus to the pan. Take the remaining sauce and re-baste the chicken and baste the asparagus as well.

Cook until the chicken reaches 165 °F.

Remove and serve!

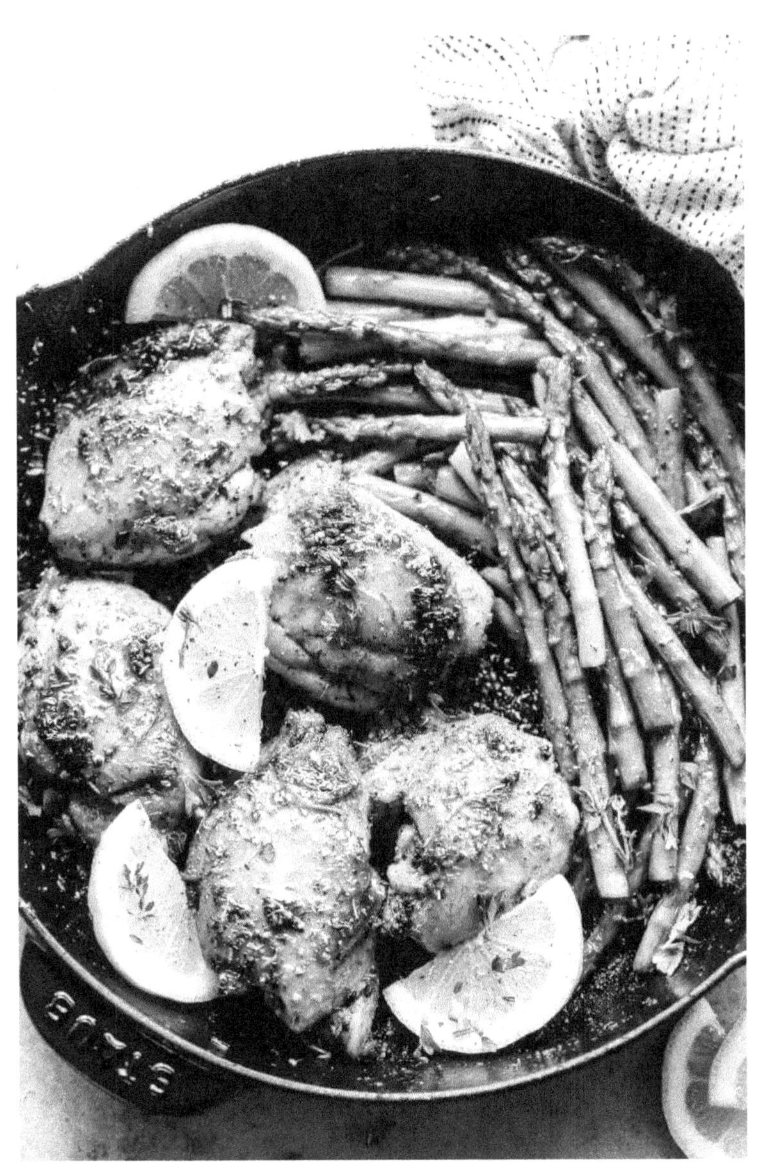

Day 7

Breakfast

Spinach and mushroom crustless quiche.

Lunch

Egg salad lettuce wraps.

Dinner

Turkey and vegetable lettuce wraps.

BREAKFAST

Spinach and mushroom crustless quiche.

INGREDIENTS

1 10oz. box frozen chopped spinach
8 oz. mushrooms
1 clove garlic, minced
1/8 tsp Salt
1 Tbsp cooking oil, divided
2 oz. feta cheese
4 large eggs
1/4 cup grated Parmesan
1/4 tsp pepper
1 cup milk
1/2 cup shredded mozzarella

INSTRUCTION

Preheat the oven to 350ºF. Thaw and squeeze as much moisture out the spinach as possible.
Rinse any dirt or debris from the mushrooms, then slice thinly.
Mince the garlic
Add the mushrooms, garlic, salt, and a ½ Tbsp cooking oil to a skillet. Sauté the mushrooms over medium heat until they have released all of their moisture and it has evaporated from the skillet. No water should remain in the skillet
Brush the other ½ Tbsp cooking oil inside a 9-inch pie plate. Layer the mushrooms, spinach, and crumbled feta into the pie plate
In a large bowl, whisk together the eggs, Parmesan, pepper, and milk

Pour the egg mixture into the pie plate over the spinach, mushrooms, and feta. Top with the shredded mozzarella
Bake the crustless quiche in the preheated 350ºF oven for about 50 minutes, or until it is golden brown on top and the internal temperature reaches 160ºF.

Slice and enjoy!

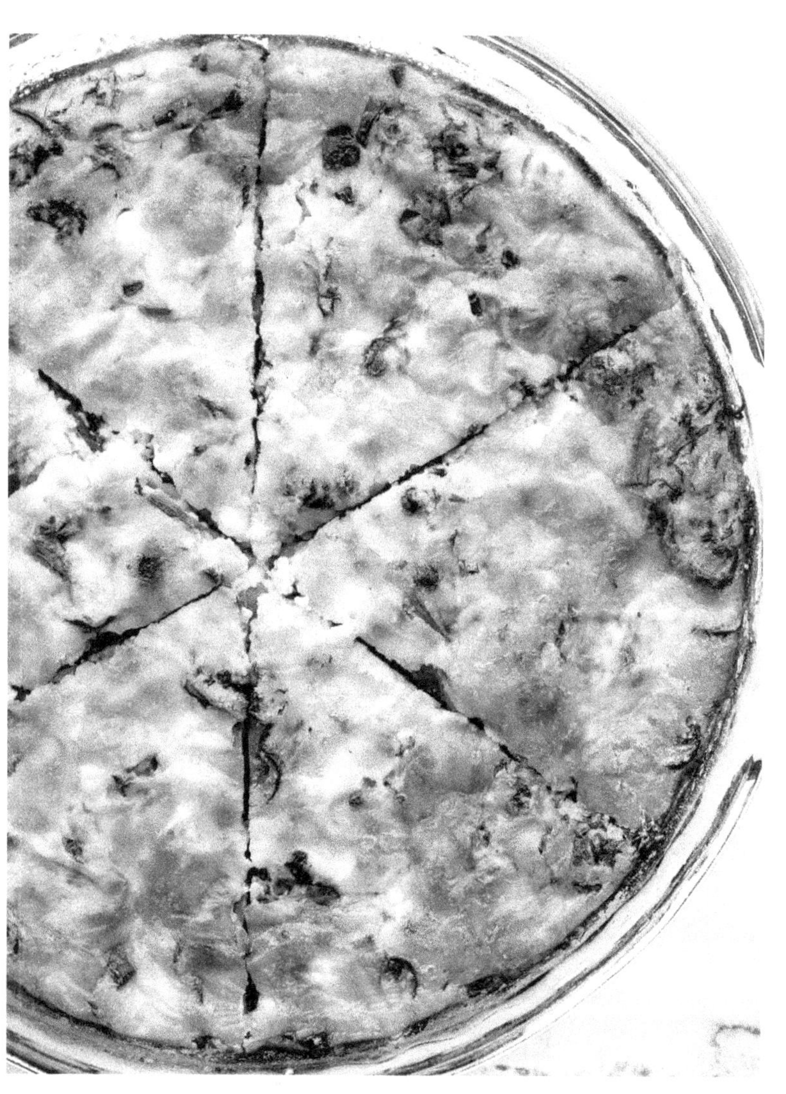

LUNCH

Egg salad lettuce wraps.

INGREDIENTS

¼ cup plain nonfat Greek yogurt
1 tablespoon mayonnaise
½ teaspoon Dijon mustard
Pinch of salt
Ground pepper to taste
3 hard-boiled eggs, peeled
2 stalks celery, minced
2 tablespoons minced red onion
2 or 3 large iceberg lettuce
leaves
1 tablespoon chopped fresh basil
2 carrots, peeled and cut into
sticks

INSTRUCTION

Whisk yogurt, mayonnaise, mustard, salt and pepper in a medium bowl. Discard one egg yolk. Chop the remaining eggs and transfer to the bowl. Add celery and onion and stir to combine. Cut lettuce leaves in half and double-layer them to make 2 lettuce wraps. Divide the egg salad among the wraps and top with basil. Serve with carrot sticks on the side.

Tips
To make ahead: Refrigerate carrot sticks and egg salad separately for up to 4 days. Chop basil and assemble lettuce wraps just before serving.

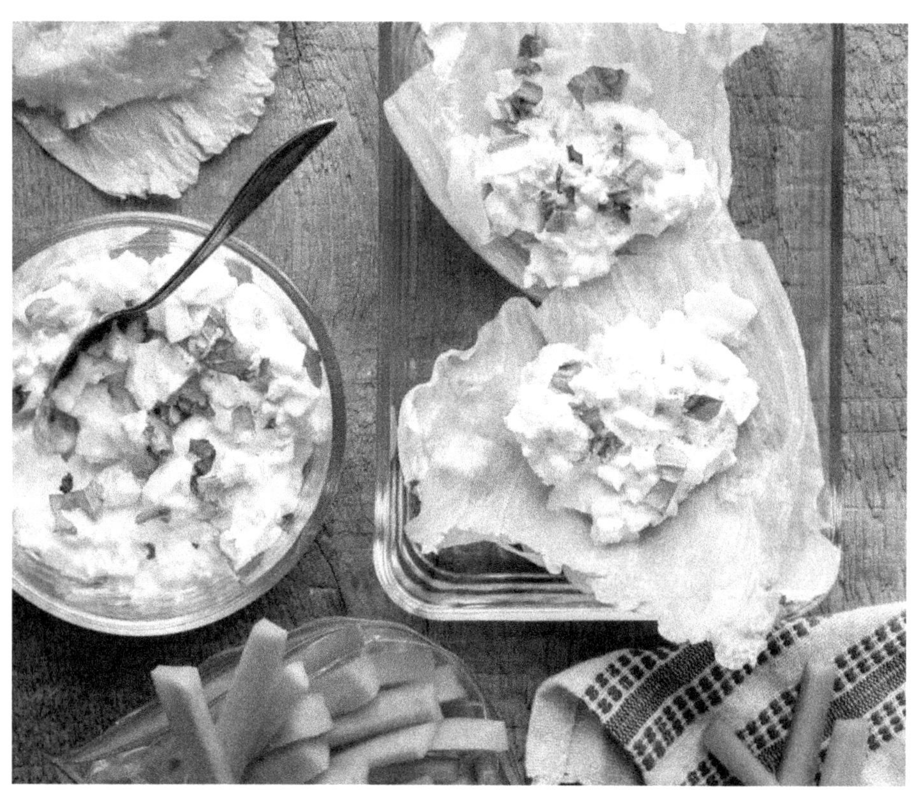

DINNER

Turkey and vegetable lettuce wraps.

INGREDIENTS

1 Pound of Ground Turkey
3-4 tablespoons Soyaki Sauce
Yellow or White Onion, chopped
3 Tablespoons of Olive Oil
1 Cup of White Rice
Cucumbers, sliced
Chopped Carrots
Cherry Tomatoes, sliced
Yellow Bell Pepper, chopped
Romain Lettuce

INSTRUCTION

Cook turkey until lightly browned
Add Soyaki to meat, set aside
Cook rice, set aside
Saute onion with olive oil and salt, set aside
Cut romain lettuce to palm sized cups
Top lettuce with rice, turkey, caramelized onions and veggies

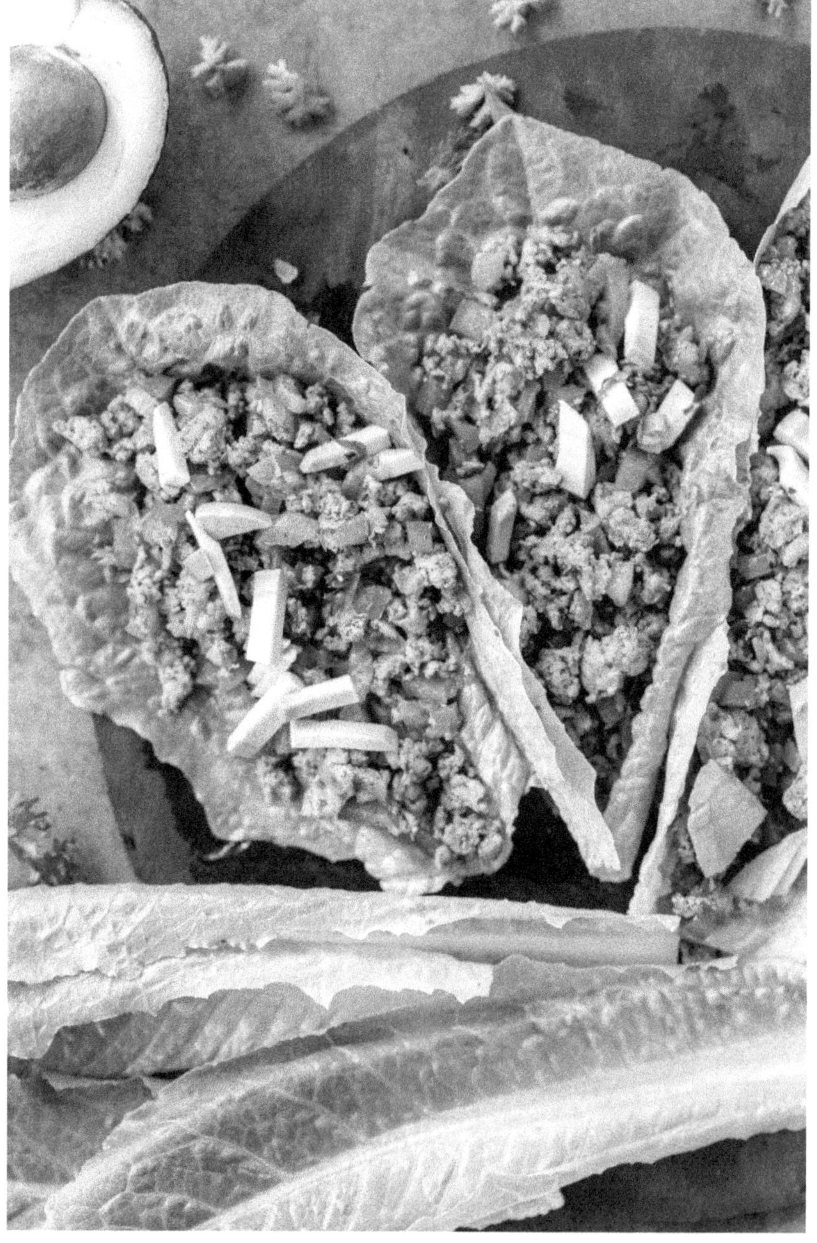

Day 8

Breakfast

Low-carb smoothie with protein powder, almond milk, and berries.

Lunch

Cauliflower fried rice with tofu and mixed vegetables.

Dinner

Eggplant lasagna with ground turkey and marinara sauce.

BREAKFAST

Low-carb smoothie with protein powder, almond milk, and berries.

INGREDIENTS

1 1/2 Cup Almond Milk
3/4 Cup Frozen Mixed Berries
1/2 tsp Vanilla Extract
2 tbsp Sweetener your preferred sweetener
1 Cup Ice

INGREDIENTS

Gather all the ingredients.

Add almond milk, frozen mixed berries, vanilla extract, sweetener and ice into a blender. Blend everything together and pour it into a cup.

Enjoy ●

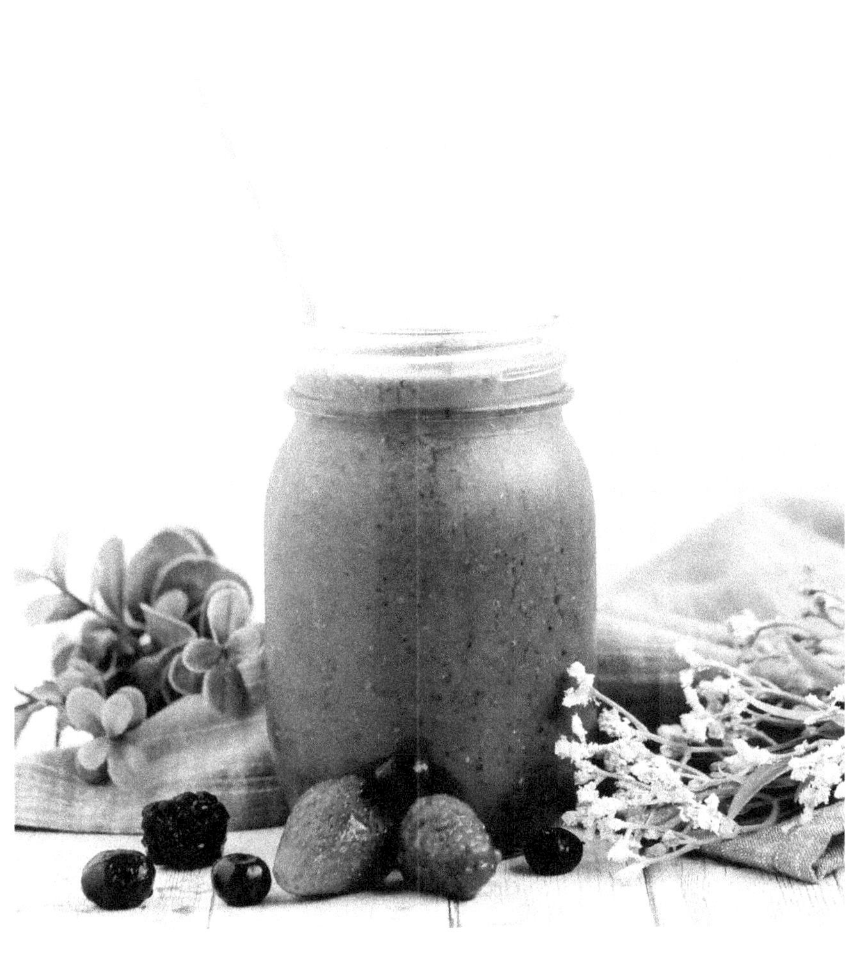

LUNCH

Cauliflower fried rice with tofu and mixed vegetables.

INGREDIENTS

Baked Tofu:
15 ounces extra firm tofu, pressed and cubed
1 tablespoon olive oil
1 tablespoon soy sauce
1 tablespoon cornstarch
Cauliflower Fried Rice:
1 medium-sized head of cauliflower, cut into florets
swish of olive oil
2 garlic cloves, minced
1 knob of ginger, grated
2–3 cups frozen peas and carrots (or really any veggies you
want)
a lil bit of soy sauce
a lil bit of Sriracha
swish of sesame oil
3 beaten eggs
green onions for topping

INGREDIENTS

Tofu: Preheat the oven to 450. Toss the tofu, olive oil, soy sauce, and cornstarch together. Arrange on a baking sheet lined with parchment paper. Bake for 20-30 minutes, stirring halfway through.

Cauliflower: Run the florets through the food processor, in batches, until they reach a rice-like consistency.

Fried "Rice": Heat your olive oil over medium heat. Add the garlic, ginger, peas, and carrots. When it's really sizzling, add the cauliflower, soy sauce, and Sriracha. Saute for just a minute or two, until the cauliflower barely softens.

Egg: Make a well in the middle of the hot pan. Add sesame oil and eggs, and gently pull the eggs around in the center with a spatula to make scrambled eggs. Once cooked, stir the scrambled eggs in with the fried rice.

Done: Serve it up, top with more Sriracha and green onions, and live your best life.

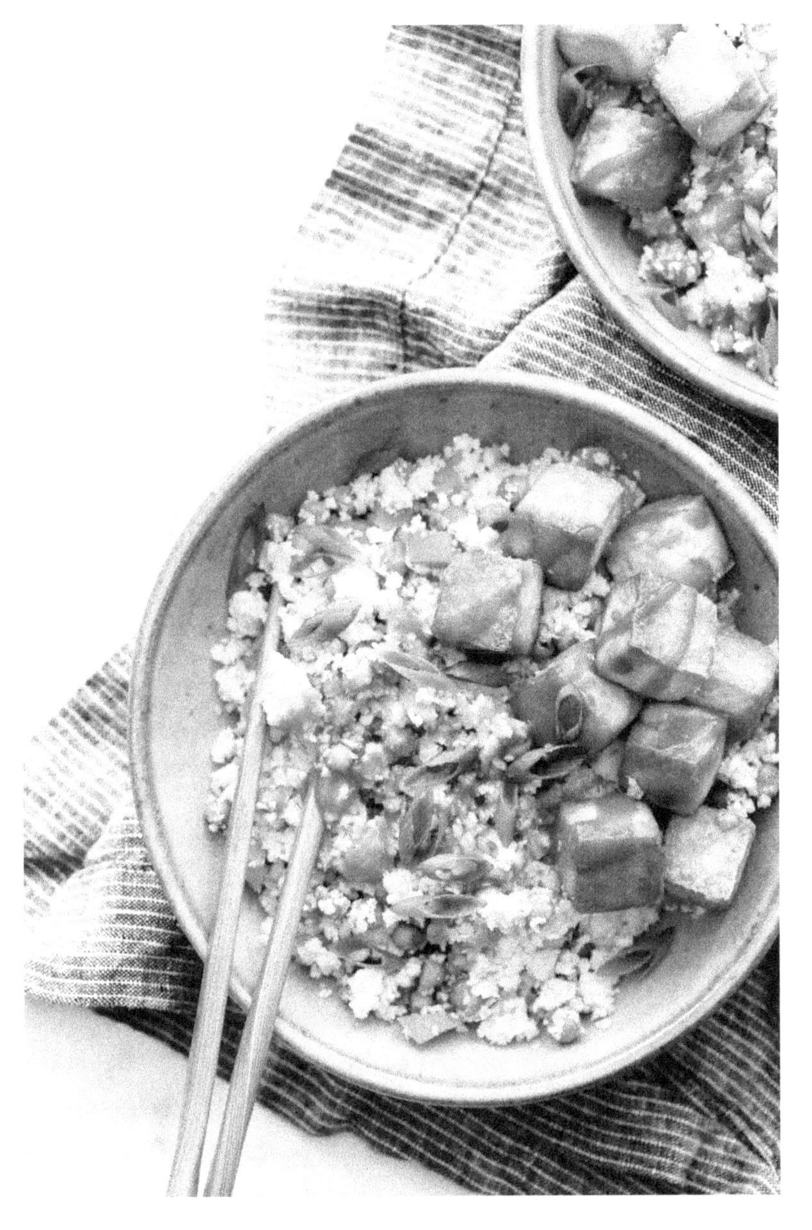

DINNER

Eggplant lasagna with ground turkey and marinara sauce.

INGREDIENTS

Eggplant lasagna with ground turkey and marinara sauce.2-3 firm eggplants, about 1 1/2 pounds (ends cut off and sliced into 12 into 1/2 inch slices cut lengthwise)

1 1/2 teaspoons salt, kosher or sea salt (divided)

4 tablespoons | 60 ml olive oil, divided

Meat Sauce

1 medium onion, diced

3 large clove | 1 heaping tablespoon garlic, minced

1 lb ground turkey

1/4 cup | 64 g tomato paste

1/2 teaspoon red chili flakes

1 teaspoon dried oregano

1 [28 oz] or 2 [14 oz] cans chopped tomatoes

2 teaspoons sugar

Cottage Cheese Filling

15 oz cottage cheese or ricotta cheese (see notes)

1 egg

1/4 cup | 22.5 grated parmesan

1 teaspoon dried parsley

1/2 teaspoon garlic powder

1/2 teaspoon freshly ground black pepper

2 cups | 226 g grated, part skim mozzarella

INSTRUCTION

Preheat oven to 400°F/205°C. Lightly grease a couple of large baking sheets.

Eggplant: Spread the eggplant slices over the prepared baking trays. Pat with a paper towel to remove surface dampness, then brush each side with 1-2 tablespoon olive oil. Spread the eggplant across the baking sheets. Leave space in-between each slice to prevent overcrowding. Sprinkle about 1/2 teaspoon salt & pepper over the top.

Place in oven and roast for 30 minutes. About halfway through, flip the eggplant and switch the baking sheets around for an even cook. When done roasting, remove the baking sheets from the oven and set aside until you're ready to assemble the lasagna.

Meat Sauce: In a large pot or skillet, add the remaining olive oil and diced onion. Cook over a medium heat for about 5-7 minutes until soft. Add the garlic and cook another minute. Add the ground turkey and cook a few minutes until no pink meat remains.

Add the tomato paste, chili flakes and oregano. Mix in and cook 2-3 minutes. Add the chopped tomatoes, sugar and salt. Let simmer and cook until a thick sauce forms, about 15-20 minutes. Stir every so often to keep the bottom from burning. Taste and season as you see fit.

Filling: In a medium-sized bowl combine the cottage cheese (or ricotta), egg, parmesan, parsley, garlic and pepper. Mix until combined.

Assemble: Lightly grease a 9in x 13in [33cm x 23cm] casserole dish. Spread about 1/2 cup of the meat sauce across the bottom of the dish. Place 6 eggplant slices evenly spread over the meat sauce. Spread half of the cottage cheese mixture over the eggplant. Sprinkle 1/2 cup mozzarella over the top. Repeat with another meat layer, the remaining eggplant, remaining cottage and another 1/2 cup of mozzarella. Spread the remaining meat sauce over the top of the casserole followed by the remaining 1 cup cheese.

Bake: Place in the middle of the oven and bake for 25-30 minutes until hot, bubbly and the cheese has turned golden. Let rest about 10 minutes before slicing and serving. Top with fresh herbs if desired and enjoy.

Notes
You can easily replace the cottage cheese with ricotta cheese for a lower fat/calorie alternative.
Make it egg free: Mixing in an egg in the ricotta/cottage cheese mixture helps make for a creamy filling that holds its shape well throughout the bake process. If you're intolerant to eggs you can simply make this without the egg - just keep in mind that the cheese layers might be more prone to slipping out as you serve this.

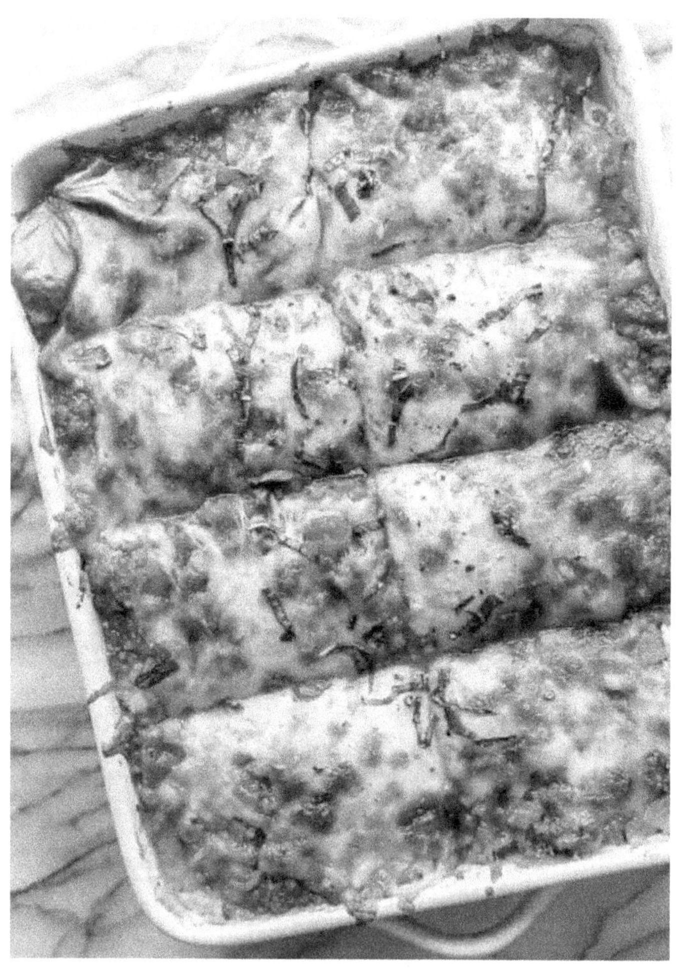

Day 9

Breakfast

Keto-friendly egg muffins with bacon and cheese.

Lunch

Caprese salad with fresh mozzarella, tomatoes, and basil.

Dinner

Spinach and feta-stuffed portobello mushrooms.

BREAKFAST

Keto-friendly egg muffins with bacon and cheese.

INGREDIENTS

6 slices bacon

nonstick cooking spray

5 eggs

½ cup shredded sharp Cheddar cheese

INSTRUCTION

Preheat the oven to 400 degrees F (200 degrees C). Line a large rimmed baking sheet with foil.

Place slices of bacon on the prepared baking sheet.

Place bacon in the preheated oven and bake until partially cooked, but still pliable, about 8 minutes. Remove from the oven, and reduce temperature to 350 degrees F (180 degrees C). Let bacon rest until cool enough to handle.

Spray 6 cups of a muffin pan with cooking spray.

Whisk eggs together in a medium bowl. Wrap a slice of bacon around the inside of each prepared muffin cup. Divide Cheddar cheese amongst the 6 muffin cups and top with beaten egg.

Bake in the oven until eggs are set, 13 to 15 minutes.

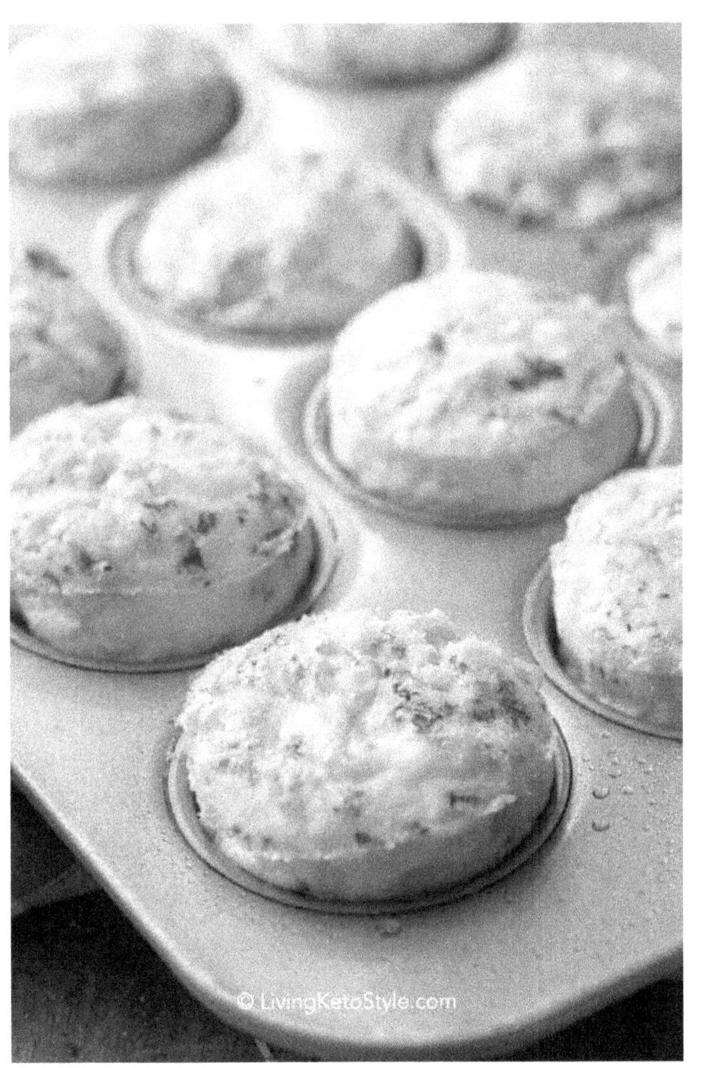
© LivingKetoStyle.com

LUNCH

Shrimp and avocado salad with lime dressing.

INGREDIENTS

1/4 cup chopped red onion
2 limes, juice of
1 tsp olive oil
1/4 tsp kosher salt, black pepper to taste
1 lb jumbo cooked, peeled shrimp, chopped*
1 medium tomato, diced
1 medium hass avocado, diced (about 5 oz)
1 jalapeno, seeds removed, diced fine
1 tbsp chopped cilantro

INSTRUCTION

In a small bowl combine red onion, lime juice, olive oil, salt and pepper. Let them marinate at least 5 minutes to mellow the flavor of the onion.

In a large bowl combine chopped shrimp, avocado, tomato, jalapeño.

Combine all the ingredients together, add cilantro and gently toss. Adjust salt and pepper to taste.

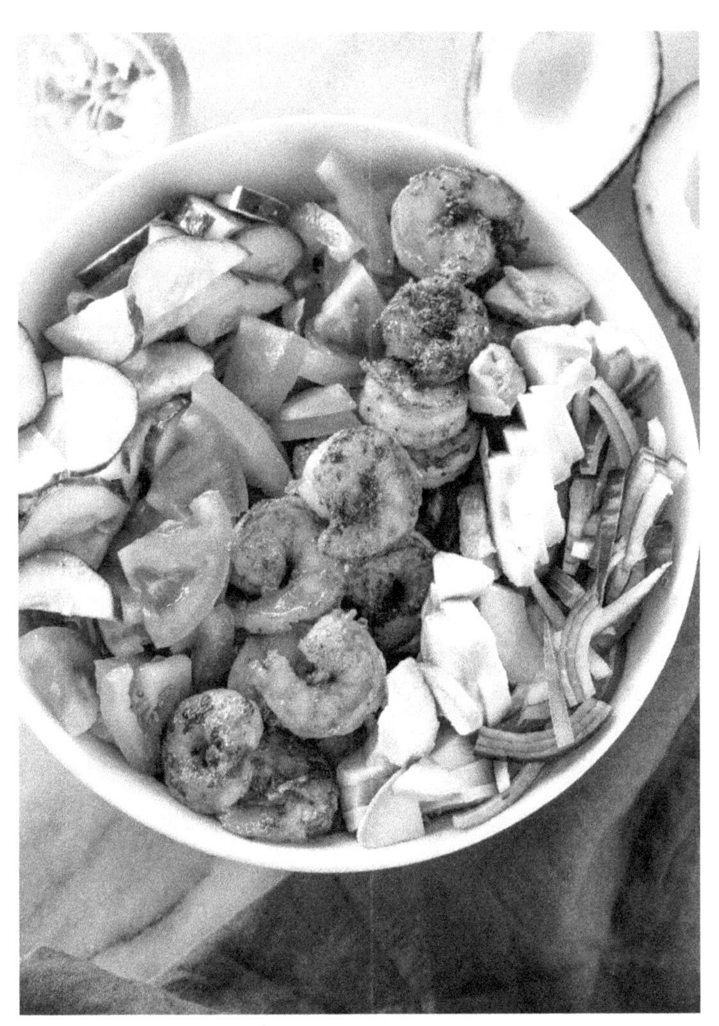

DINNER

Spinach and feta-stuffed portobello mushrooms

INGREDIENTS

3 tablespoons extra-virgin olive oil, divided
1 bunch scallions, sliced
2 cloves garlic, minced
1 (10 ounce) package frozen chopped spinach, thawed and
squeezed dry
½ cup crumbled feta cheese, plus 1 tablespoon
¼ cup chopped fresh dill
¼ teaspoon ground pepper
⅛ teaspoon salt
4 medium portobello mushrooms, stems and gills removed (see Tip)
Crushed red pepper for garnish

INSTRUCTION

Preheat oven to 400 degrees F.

Heat 2 tablespoons oil in a large skillet over medium heat. Add
scallions and garlic; cook, stirring, until softened, about 3 minutes.
Remove from heat and stir in spinach, 1/2 cup feta, dill, pepper and
salt.

Brush mushrooms all over with the remaining 1 tablespoon oil.
Place on a baking sheet and divide the spinach mixture among the
mushrooms. Bake until hot and starting to brown, 15 to 20 minutes.
Sprinkle with the remaining 1 tablespoon feta and with crushed red
pepper, if desired, and serve.

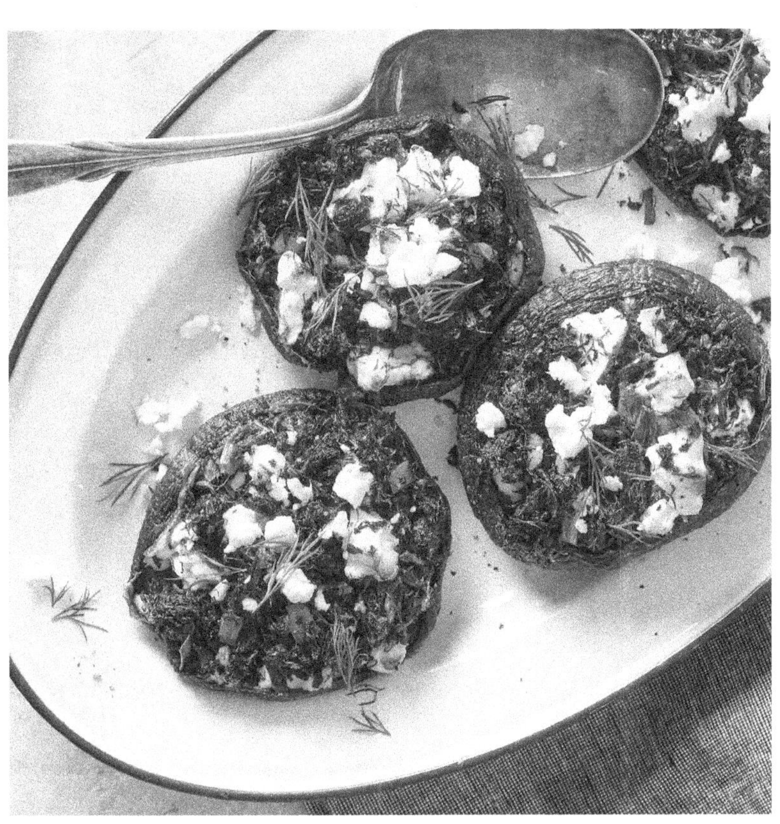

Day 10

Breakfast

Almond flour pancakes with sugar-free syrup.

Lunch

Tuna salad with avocado and cucumber slices.

Dinner

Cabbage and ground beef stir-fry with ginger and garlic.

BREAKFAST

Almond flour pancakes with sugar-free syrup.

INGREDIENTS

2 cups almond flour
1 tsp baking powder
1/4 tsp salt
2 eggs
1/2 cup unsweetened almond milk
2 tbsp coconut oil, melted
1 tsp vanilla extract
1/4 cup sugar-free maple syrup

INSTRUCTION

In a bowl, mix together the almond flour, baking powder, and salt.

Add in the eggs, almond milk, coconut oil, and vanilla extract. Stir until fully combined.

Heat a non-stick pan over medium heat. Scoop 1/4 cup of batter onto the pan and cook until bubbles form on top, then flip and cook until golden brown.

Repeat until all the batter is used up.

Serve with sugar-free maple syrup.

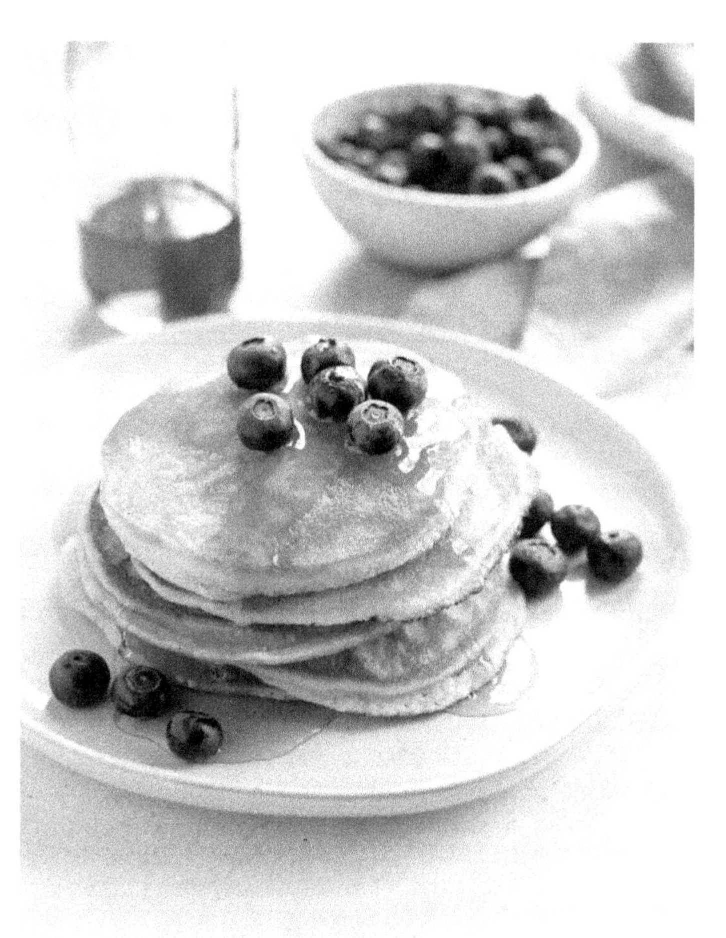

LUNCH

Tuna salad with avocado and cucumber slices.

INGREDIENTS

3 cans (5-ounces each) tuna in water, drained and
flaked
2 large avocados, peeled, pitted, and cut into a larger
dice
1 English cucumber, sliced into half moons
1 small red onion, thinly sliced
¼ cup chopped parsley or cilantro
¼ cup olive oil
juice of 1 lemon
salt and fresh ground pepper, to taste

INSTRUCTION

Place prepped tuna into a large salad bowl.

Add in diced avocado, cucumber slices, sliced onions, and parsley
or cilantro. Set aside.

In a small mixing bowl combine olive oil, lemon juice, salt, and
pepper; whisk to combine.

Taste for seasonings and adjust accordingly. I almost always add
more lemon and salt.

Add salad dressing to the salad; toss to combine.

Serve.

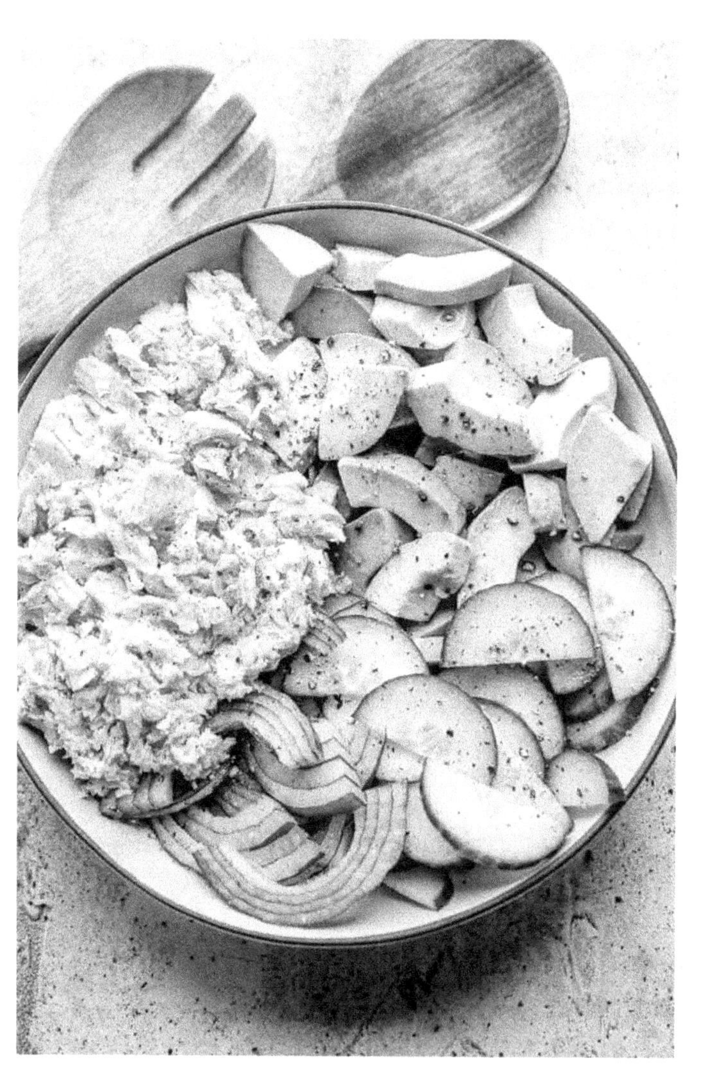

DINNER

Cabbage and ground beef stir-fry with ginger and garlic.

INGREDIENTS

1 pound grass-fed ground beef like Moink

¼ teaspoon salt

½ medium onion diced

3 cloves garlic minced

3 Tablespoons freshly minced ginger

1 head green cabbage about 10-12 cups shredded

2 Tablespoons tamari or gluten-free soy sauce

¼ teaspoon red pepper flakes

1 teaspoon sesame oil

optional: green onion for garnish

1 cup brown rice + 2 cups water

INSTRUCTION

Heat a large pan or wok over medium-high heat. Add the beef, season with a little salt, and brown on all sides, stirring to break up the meat. If using extra lean beef, you may need a little oil in the pan.

Meanwhile, chop up an onion into medium dice. Once beef is mostly browned, add the diced onions and sauté about 5 minutes.

Stir in the minced garlic and ginger and cook for another 30 seconds, then add the cabbage, soy sauce, and red pepper flakes. Stir fry (uncovered) until cabbage is wilted and soft. Remove from heat. Drizzle with 1 teaspoon sesame oil and sprinkle with chopped green onion for serving.

Enjoy as is or with brown rice.

For brown rice: prepare in rice cooker if available, or follow package instructions. Add 1 cup uncooked brown rice to a large pot with 2 cups of water and bring to a boil. Reduce to a simmer and cook about 40 minutes. Remove from heat (without removing lid!), and set aside to steam for 10 minutes. Fluff with a fork and serve.

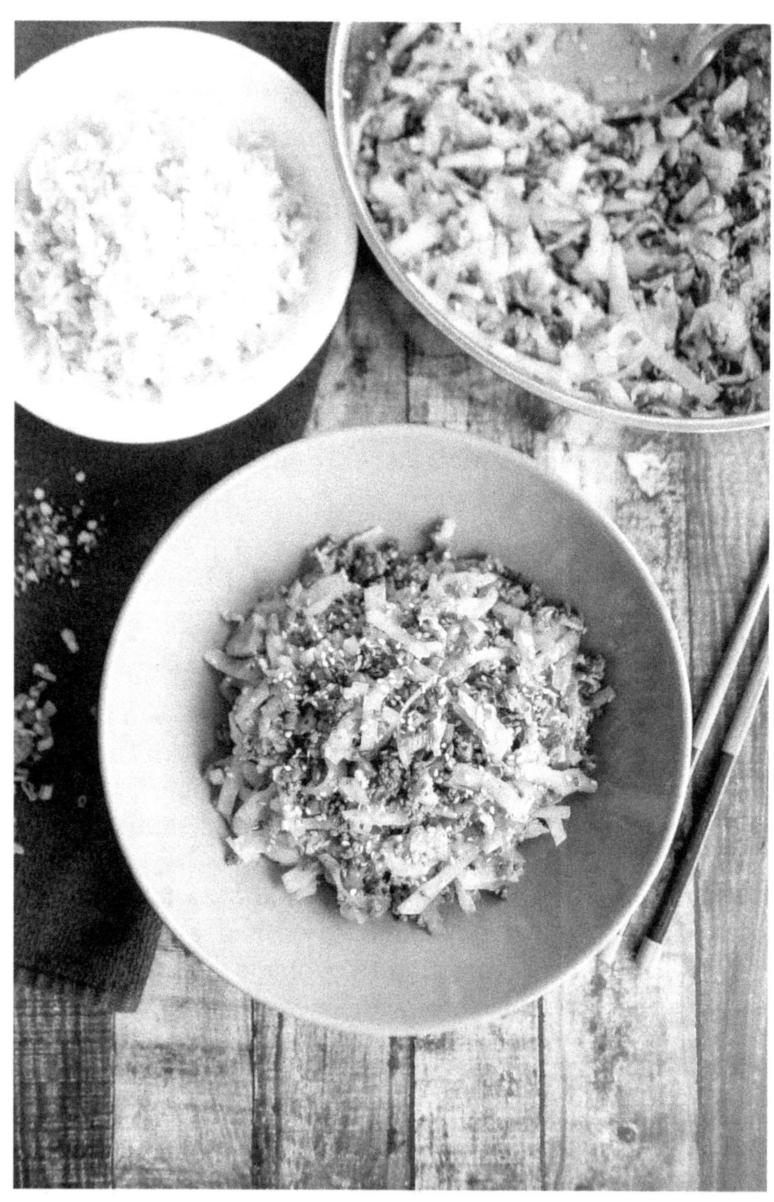

Day 11

Breakfast

Veggie and cheese-stuffed bell peppers.

Lunch

Grilled salmon with asparagus and lemon.

Dinner

Keto-friendly taco salad with ground beef, lettuce, and cheese.

BREAKFAST

Veggie and cheese-stuffed bell peppers.

INGREDIENTS

4 large red bell peppers, halved from stem to base, seeds and
membranes removed

1 tablespoon extra virgin olive oil, as needed

Fine salt and freshly ground black pepper, for sprinkling

Filling and topping

½ cup long-grain brown rice (or 1 ½ cups cooked rice)

2 tablespoons extra virgin olive oil

1 large yellow onion, chopped

½ teaspoon fine salt, to taste

1 pint (2 cups) cherry tomatoes, halved or quartered if large

½ cup chopped fresh cilantro, plus more for garnish

4 cloves garlic, pressed or minced

1 ½ teaspoons chili powder

1 teaspoon ground cumin

1 can (1 ½ cups) pinto beans, rinsed and drained

Freshly ground black pepper, to taste

1 tablespoon lime juice

4 ounces (about 1 cup) grated part-skim mozzarella or cheddar

Optional garnishes: Sliced ripe avocado or guacamole, perhaps
a drizzle of cilantro-hemp pesto, red salsa, sour cream or vegan
sour cream

INSTRUCTION

To roast the peppers: Preheat the oven to 425 degrees Fahrenheit. Place the halved peppers in a large 9 by 13-inch baking dish, or on a rimmed baking sheet lined with parchment paper. Drizzle 1 tablespoon olive oil over the peppers and sprinkle them with salt and pepper. Use your hands to rub the oil all over both sides of the peppers, then arrange them with the cut sides facing up. Bake for 20 to 25 minutes, until the peppers are a little blistered around the edges and easily pierced through by a fork. Set aside. Leave the oven on for baking the peppers.

In the meantime, cook the rice: Bring a large pot of water to boil. Rinse the rice in a fine-mesh colander until the water runs clear. Add the rice to the boiling water and continue boiling, uncovered, for 30 minutes (reduce the heat as necessary to prevent overflow). Drain off the remaining cooking water and return the rice to the pot. Set aside.

Prepare the filling: In a large skillet over medium heat, warm 2 tablespoons olive oil until shimmering. Add the onion and ½ teaspoon of the salt. Cook, stirring often, until the onion is tender, about 5 minutes. Add the tomatoes and cook until they're lightly squishy, another 5 minutes or so.

Add the cilantro, garlic, chili powder and cumin. While stirring, cook until the garlic is fragrant, about 30 to 60 seconds.

Remove the pot from the heat and add the rice, beans, lime juice and about 10 twists of black pepper. Stir to combine, then season with additional salt (I usually add ¼ teaspoon) and black pepper, to taste.

To stuff the peppers, first pour off any excess juice pooled within the peppers. Then stuff each pepper generously with the rice mixture (if the peppers were truly large, you should have just the right amount of filling—if you have extra, save it to serve as a side dish). Top the peppers with the cheese.

Bake at 425 for 12 to 13 minutes, until the cheese is golden in spots. Serve warm with fresh cilantro leaves on top or any other garnishes of your choice. Leftovers keep well in the fridge, covered, for up to 4 days. I believe they would freeze well for several months, but haven't tried to be sure.

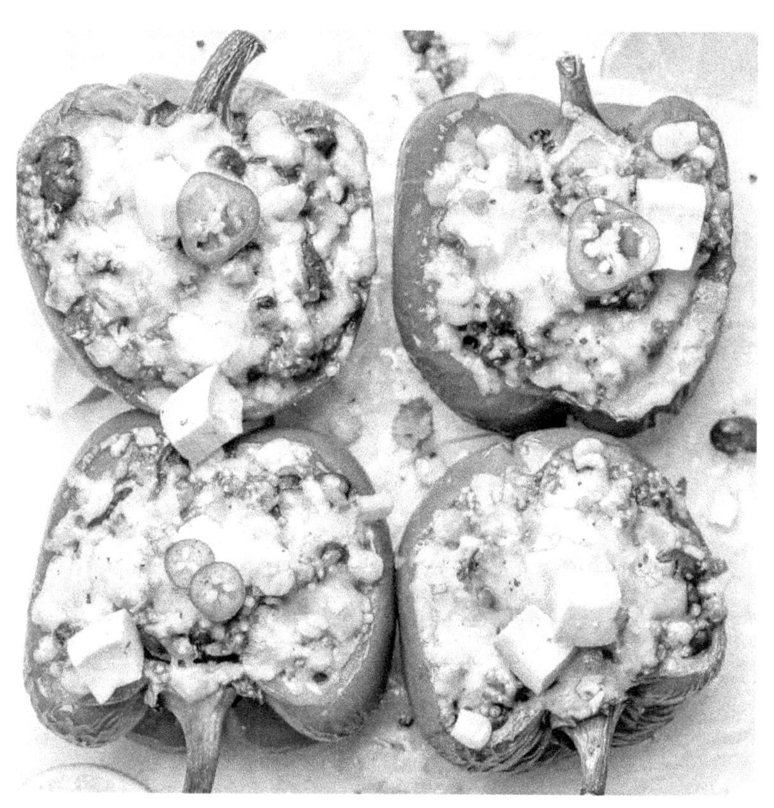

LUNCH

Grilled salmon with asparagus and lemon.

INGREDIENTS

20 asparagus spears, trimmed
4 6-oz. skin-on salmon fillets
4 tbsp. butter, divided
2 lemons, sliced
kosher salt
Freshly ground black pepper
Torn fresh dill, for garnish

INSTRUCTION

Step 1
Lay two pieces of foil on a flat surface. Place five spears of asparagus on foil and top with a fillet of salmon, 1 tablespoon butter, and two slices lemon. Loosely wrap, then repeat with remaining ingredients until you have four packets total.

Step 2
Heat grill on high. Add foil packets to grill and grill until salmon is cooked through and asparagus is tender, about 10 minutes.

Step 3
Garnish with dill and serve.

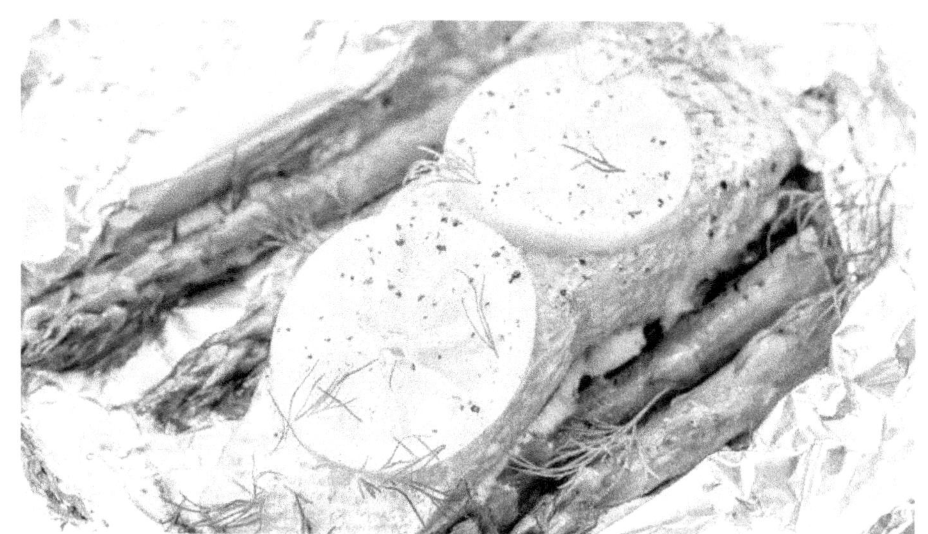

DINNER

Keto-friendly taco salad with ground beef,
lettuce, and cheese.

INGREDIENTS

1 1/2 pounds of lean ground beef

2 tablespoons of cooking oil

1 medium green bell pepper chopped finely

1 medium onion finely chopped

1 teaspoon of onion powder

3/4 teaspoon of garlic powder

1 teaspoon of chili powder

3/4 teaspoon of cumin powder

1/2 teaspoon of chipotle pepper

1/2 teaspoon of black pepper

1 1/4 teaspoon of salt

3 hearts of Romaine lettuce, torn into bite sizes

2 cups of grape tomatoes, sliced in half

1 cup of Mexican blend shredded cheddar cheese or shredded
cheddar cheese

2 medium Hass avocado, diced

1/2 a cup of red onions, sliced

1/2 cup of green onions, sliced

2 tablespoons of chopped cilantro (garnish)

1/4 cup of sliced black olives

Creamy Salsa Dressing

1 cup salsa

1 cup sour cream thinned with two tablespoons of heavy cream
or Mexican crema

1/4 teaspoon of onion powder

1/4 teaspoon of garlic powder

1/4 teaspoon of cumin powder

1/4 teaspoon of chili powder

1/4 teaspoon of black pepper

1/4 teaspoon of chipotle pepper

1/4 teaspoon of salt

INSTRUCTION

Over medium-high heat, in a large skillet cook, the bell peppers and onions with the two tablespoons of cooking oil until translucent then set them aside.

Turn the stove to high and add the ground beef to the skillet. Then sprinkle all the dry seasonings and cook the meat until brown being sure to break it into pieces with a spatula until cooked.

Stir in the cooked bell peppers and onions to the cooked ground beef and set it aside.

Proceed to make the creamy salsa dressing.

Creamy Salsa Dressing

In a small bowl combine the salsa, Mexican crema, or sour cream that has been thinned with two tablespoons of heavy cream, and dry spices. Mix well until it is well incorporated. Set it aside.

Assembling The Salad

Note that the salad can be served individually or in a large bowl. Place the torn lettuce in a large bowl or serving tray as the bottom layer. Then arrange the halved tomatoes, cheddar cheese, black olives, avocados, green onions, and red onions, on top of the lettuce.

Place the cooked taco meat on top of the salad. Garnish with chopped fresh cilantro.

Toss the salad and serve the salsa dressing on the side.

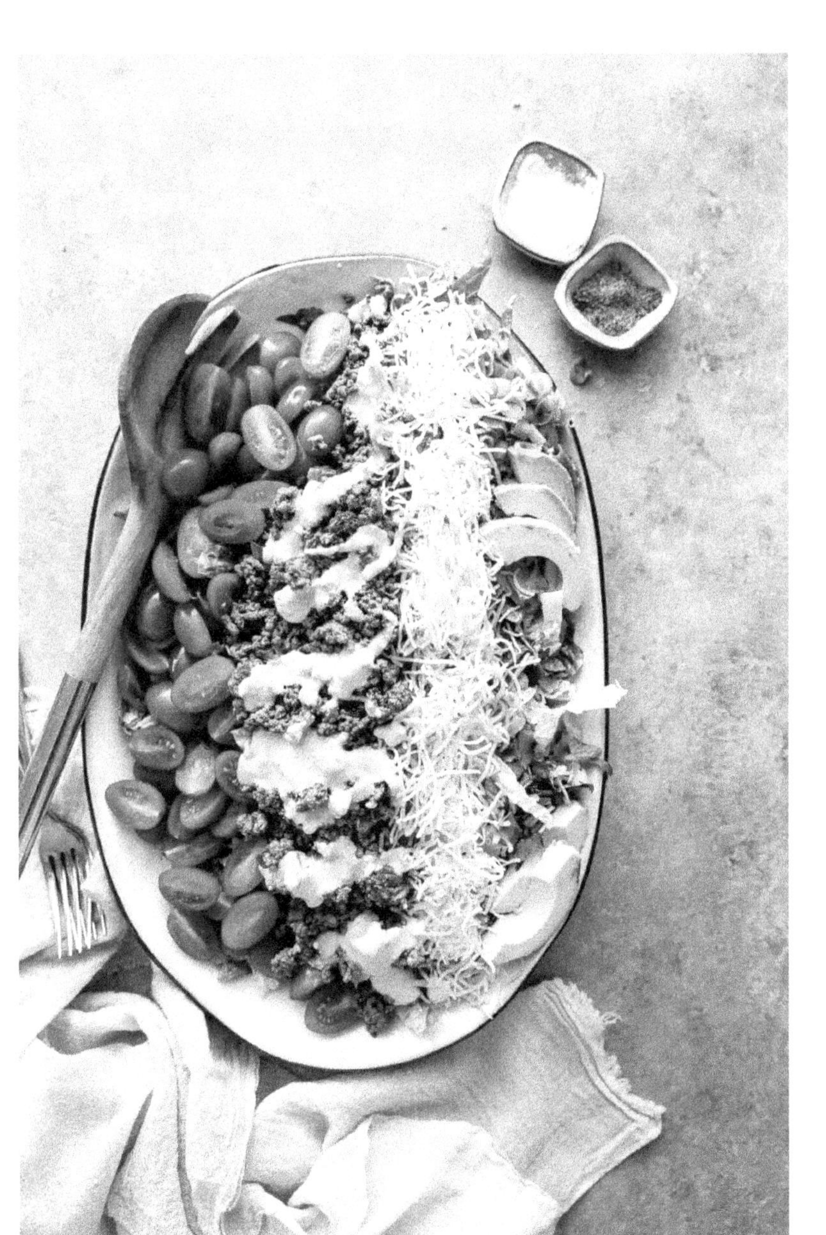

Day 12

Breakfast

Smoked turkey and cheese roll-ups.

Lunch

Shrimp and avocado salad with lime dressing.

Dinner

Baked cod with lemon and dill, paired with roasted broccoli.

BREAKFAST

Smoked turkey and cheese roll-ups.

INGREDIENTS

4 ounces low-fat cream cheese
4 green onions, chopped
1/2 cup cucumber, seeded and chopped
1/2 teaspoon dill weed
4 flour tortillas
4 ounces smoked turkey

INSTRUCTION

Combine cream cheese with onions, cucumber and dill weed.

Spread each tortilla with 1/4 of the mixture, top with some smoked turkey and roll up.

The rolls may also be sliced across to make appetizers.

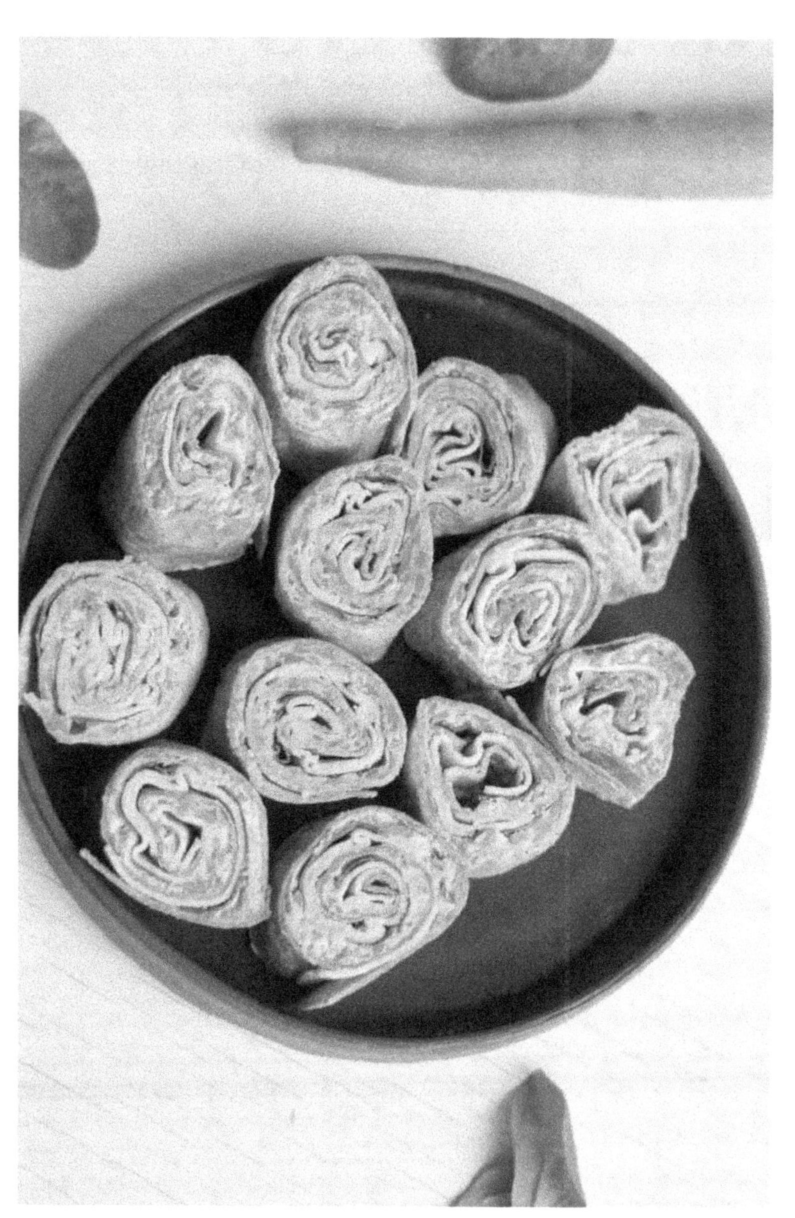

LUNCH

Shrimp and avocado salad with lime dressing.

INGREDIENTS

1/4 cup chopped red onion
2 limes, juice of
1 tsp olive oil
1/4 tsp kosher salt, black pepper to taste
1 lb jumbo cooked, peeled shrimp, chopped*
1 medium tomato, diced
1 medium hass avocado, diced (about 5 oz)
1 jalapeno, seeds removed, diced fine
1 tbsp chopped cilantro

INSTRUCTION

In a small bowl combine red onion, lime juice, olive oil, salt and pepper. Let them marinate at least 5 minutes to mellow the flavor of the onion.

In a large bowl combine chopped shrimp, avocado, tomato, jalapeño.

Combine all the ingredients together, add cilantro and gently toss. Adjust salt and pepper to taste.

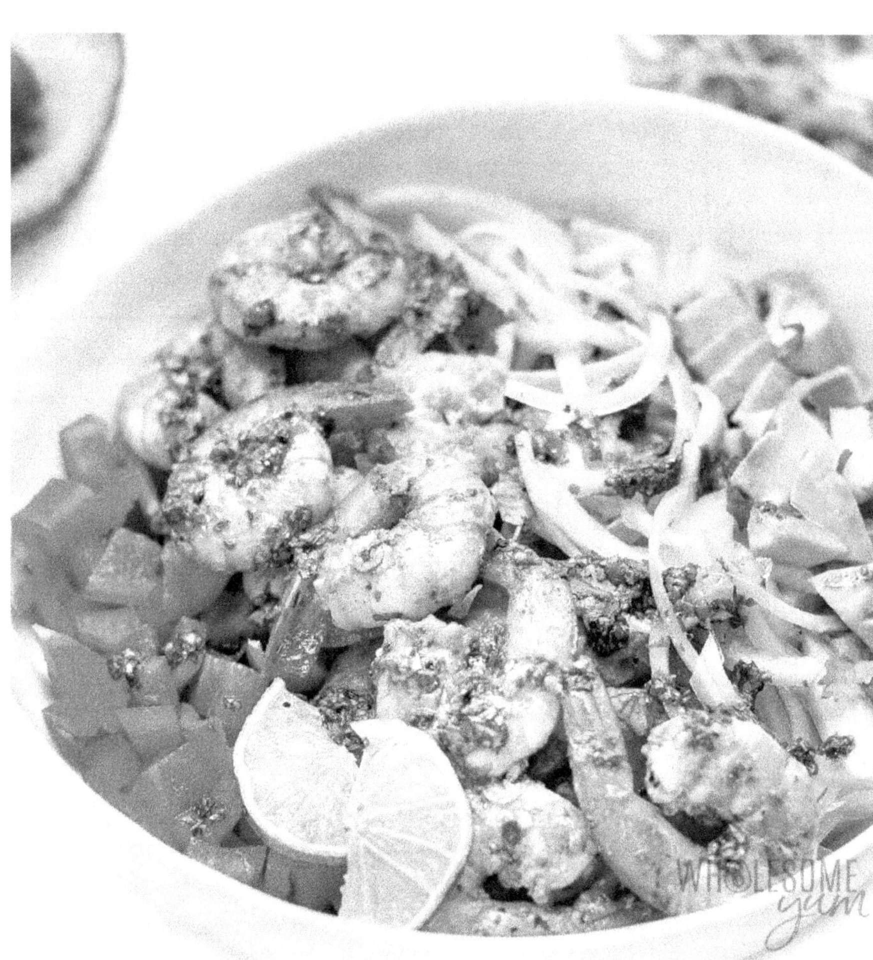

DINNER

Baked cod with lemon and dill, paired with roasted broccoli.

INGREDIENTS

8 4-oz Cod fillets (preferably thawed)
1/4 cup Unsalted butter
1 medium Lemon (juiced and zested; see notes*)
1/2 tsp Garlic powder
3/4 tsp Sea salt
1/4 tsp Black pepper
1 tbsp Fresh parsley (chopped)

INSTRUCTION

Preheat the oven to 400 degrees F (204 degrees C). You can bake the cod fillets from frozen or thaw them first in a bowl of cold water. (I prefer thawing if you have time, as it makes it easier to brush on the butter without solidifying.)

Use paper towels to pat the cod fillets dry. Arrange them in a single layer in a 9×13 baking dish.

In a small bowl in the microwave or saucepan on the stove, melt the butter. Remove from heat. Stir in the lemon juice and lemon zest.

Brush the lemon butter over the cod fillets. Season with garlic powder, sea salt, and black pepper. Flip and repeat both lemon butter and seasoning on the other side.

Bake for 12-15 minutes (will vary by thickness), until the baked cod is opaque and flakes easily with a fork. Sprinkle with fresh parsley and serve.

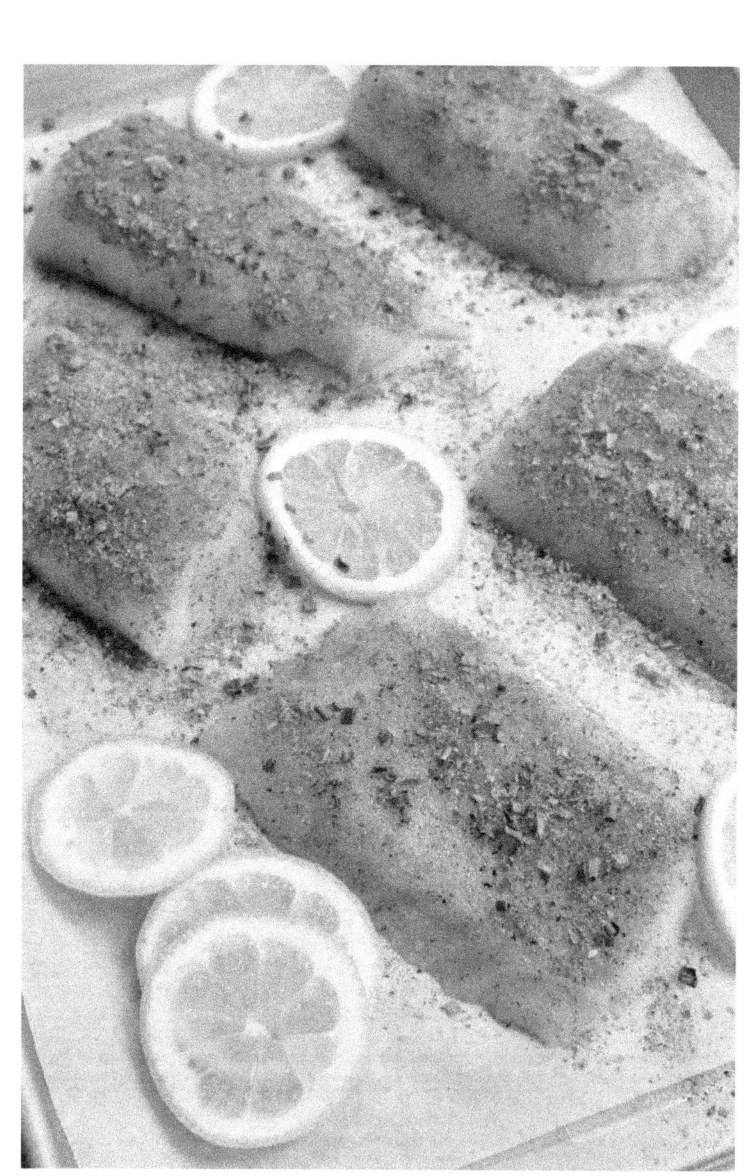

Day 13

Breakfast

Broccoli and cheddar frittata.

Lunch

Chicken and vegetable skewers with tzatziki sauce.

Dinner

Stuffed bell peppers with ground turkey, cauliflower rice, and spices.

Breakfast

Broccoli and cheddar frittata.

INGREDIENTS

1 tbsp olive oil, extra virgin
2 cups broccoli, chopped
1/2 white or yellow onion, diced
8 eggs
1/2 cup milk of choice
1 cup shredded cheddar cheese, can use
mozzarella or a four cheese blend
1 tsp salt
1/2 tsp garlic powder
1/4 tsp ground mustard
1/4 tsp cayenne pepper
1/4 tsp black pepper

INSTRUCTION

Preheat the oven to 425 degrees.

Heat oil in a cast iron skillet on medium to medium-high heat.

Once hot, add chopped broccoli and onion. Sauté until tender, stirring frequently, 3 to 5 minutes.

Meanwhile, whisk together the eggs, milk, salt, garlic powder, ground mustard, cayenne pepper, and black pepper. When the broccoli and onion are done, turn off the stove.

Spread the broccoli and onion mixture across the bottom of the skillet so they're evenly distributed. Layer the shredded cheese on top. Pour your egg mixture over everything.

Bake until the center is just set, 12 to 15 minutes. Check to make sure the center isn't very wiggly and then remove from the oven. Let it rest for a few minutes before serving. The frittata will bubble a lot in the oven and settle down as it rests.

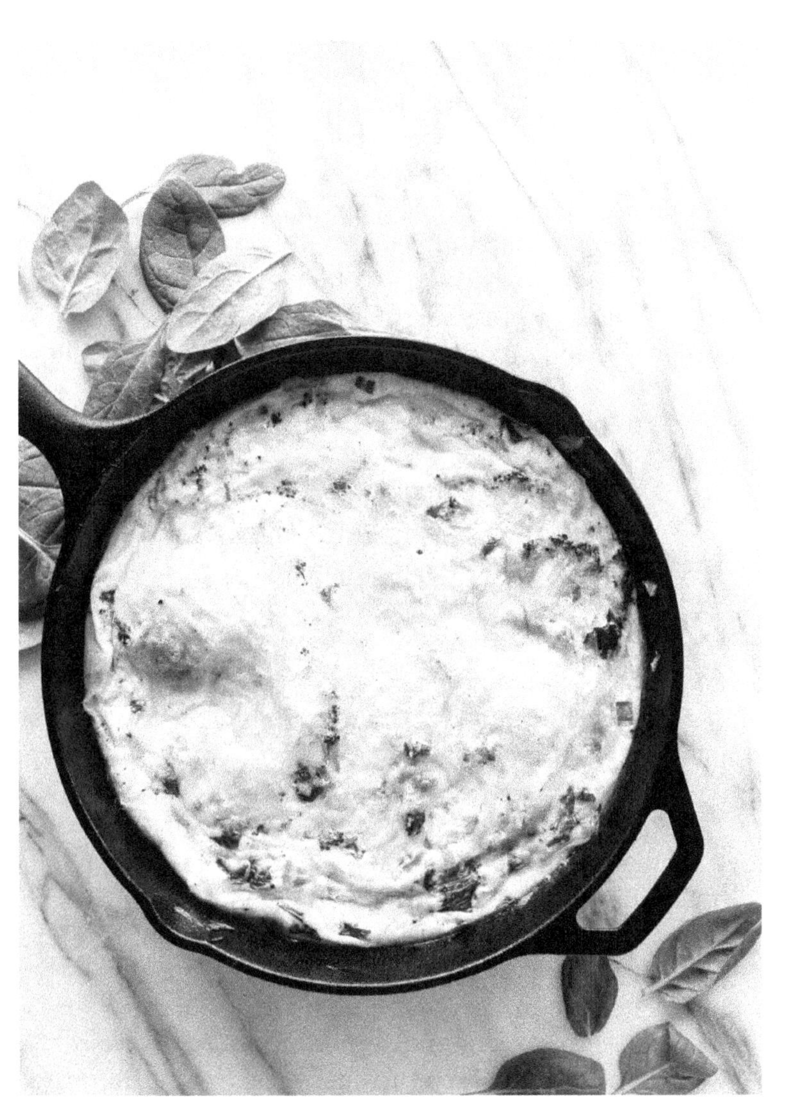

LUNCH

Chicken and vegetable skewers with tzatziki sauce.

INGREDIENTS

2 tablespoons olive oil
1 lemon, juiced
1 tablespoon dried oregano
½ teaspoon garlic powder
½ teaspoon salt
4 boneless skinless chicken thighs, cut into 1" pieces
1 small zucchini, sliced into 1/4" moons
1 red onion, chopped
14 cherry tomatoes
½ cup prepared tzatziki, store-bought or recipe as follows
Tzatziki Sauce
½ cup Greek yogurt
¼ cucumber, seeds removed & chopped fine
1 tablespoon chopped fresh mint
2 cloves garlic, finely minced
¼ teaspoon salt

INSTRUCTION

Mix the olive oil, lemon juice, oregano, garlic powder, and 1/2 teaspoon salt together in a bowl. Add the chicken and toss to coat. Set aside for 30 minutes (up to 2 hours) to marinate, tossing occasionally.
To make the tzatziki (can be made ahead):
Remove excess moisture from the chopped cucumber by blotting with a towel. Place the cucumber, Greek yogurt, mint, garlic, and salt in a small bowl and mix to combine.
Cover & store in your cooler if making ahead of time.
Prepare a grill or campfire for grilling.
Thread the chicken and vegetables onto skewers.
Once the grill is ready, place the skewers on the grill grate and grill, turning every few minutes so all sides cook evenly. The chicken will need to cook 3-5 minutes per side, and the veggies will need roughly 10-12 minutes.
Remove skewers. Serve with tzatziki for dipping. Enjoy!

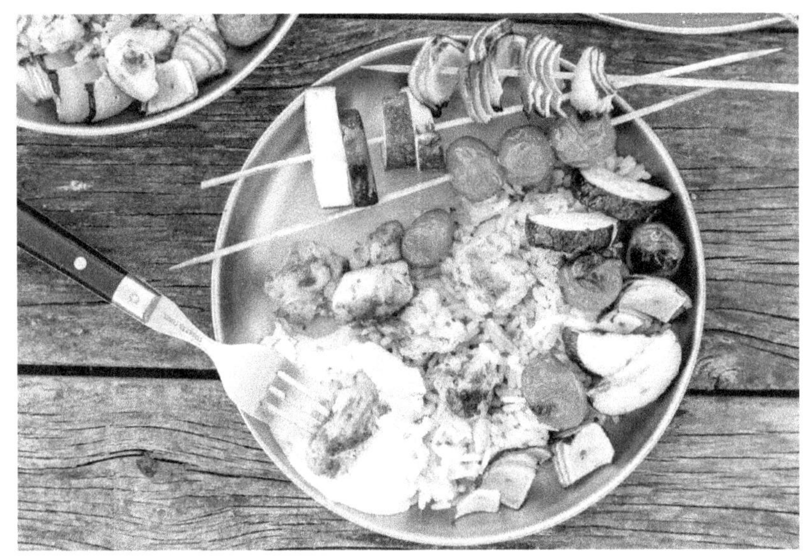

DINNER

Stuffed bell peppers with ground turkey, cauliflower rice, and spices.

INGREDIENTS

FOR THE MARINARA SAUCE:

1 Can (28 ounces) Whole Peeled Tomatoes (nothing beats San Marzano)
1 Medium Sized Onion, diced
3 LARGE Cloves Garlic, chopped
1 Tablespoon Olive Oil
1 teaspoon ea Dried Oregano, Sea Salt and Sugar
Pinch of Red Pepper Flakes
5-6 Fresh Basil Leaves, chopped

FOR THE FILLING:

6 Bell Peppers, tops chopped off, rims and seeds removed
2 Tablespoons Olive Oil, divided
1 lb. Ground Turkey
¾ Cup Onion, diced
3 Cloves Garlic, minced
1 teaspoon ea Cumin, Chili Powder, Sea Salt
¼ teaspoon Black Pepper
1 ½ Cups Mariana Sauce (see below)
2 Cups Cauliflower Rice (see below)
Monterey Jack Cheese

INSTRUCTION

Prepare the Cauliflower Rice: Trim the cauliflower florets and pulse them in a food processor until they resemble couscous. Toss with olive oil, sea salt, and black pepper. Spread on a baking sheet and bake at 350°F for 15 minutes. Set aside to cool.

Make the Marinara Sauce: In a medium saucepan, sauté diced onions in olive oil until softened. Add garlic, tomatoes, oregano, salt, sugar, and red pepper flakes. Simmer for 30-45 minutes, occasionally crushing the tomatoes with a spoon. Remove from heat, discard the onion, and pulse the sauce in a food processor for desired consistency. Stir in chopped basil.

Prepare the Filling: Sauté diced onion, ground turkey, and garlic in olive oil until the turkey is browned and cooked through. Add cumin, chili powder, salt, and pepper. Combine with cauliflower rice and 1 ½ cups of marinara sauce. Stir in approximately 1 cup of cheese.

Stuff the Peppers: Spoon the filling into each bell pepper, adding chunks of cheese if desired. Place the stuffed peppers in a loaf pan, pour about ¼ cup of water in each pan, cover with aluminum foil, and bake at 350°F for 30-45 minutes or until peppers are soft and easily pierced with a knife.

Serve and Enjoy: Let the stuffed peppers cool for 5-10 minutes before serving. Savor the delightful flavors of seasoned turkey and cauliflower rice, complemented by the rich and comforting marinara sauce. These stuffed peppers are perfect for a hearty weeknight dinner or for preparing ahead and freezing for later enjoyment.

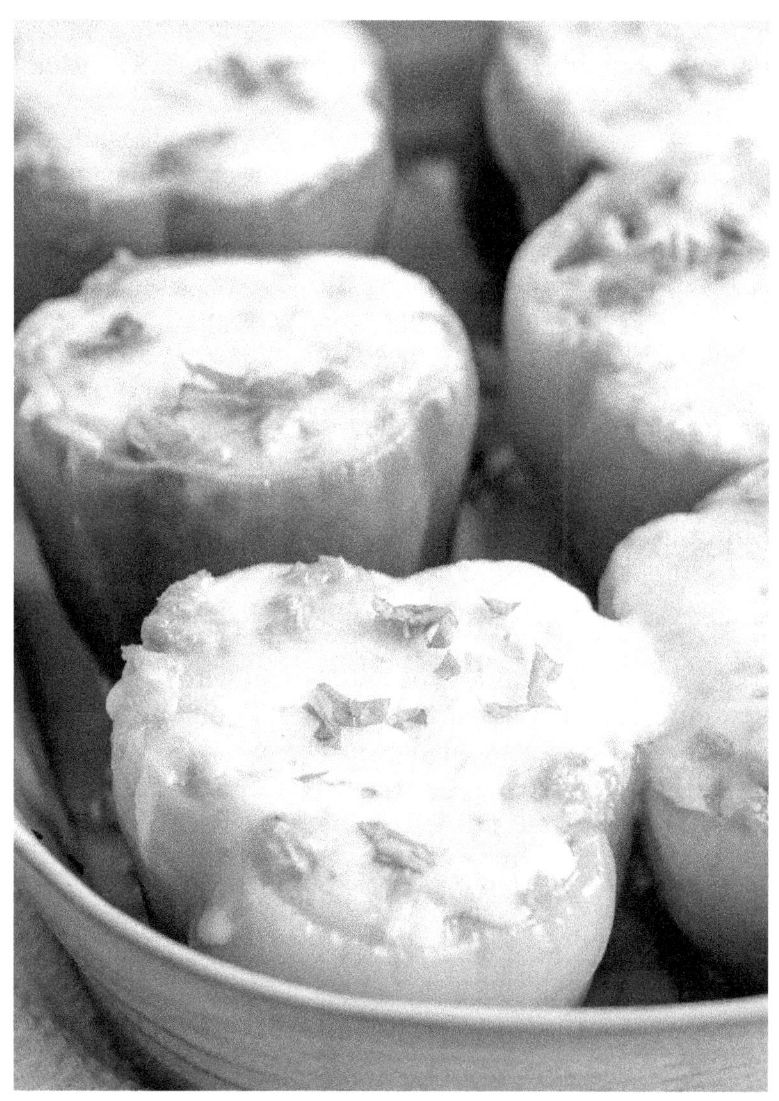

Day 14

Breakfast

Keto avocado and bacon egg cups.

Lunch

Creamy cauliflower soup with bacon and cheddar.

Dinner

Spinach and bacon salad with a creamy dressing.

Breakfast

Keto avocado and bacon egg cups.

INGREDIENTS

6 rashers bacon
3 small avocados or 2 large
3 tsp hot sauce or to taste
salt and pepper
squeeze of lemon juice
6 eggs free run

INSTRUCTION

Pre heat the oven to 220ºc / 430ºf
Line each muffin mould with bacon - I used a small piece to lay on the bottom of the tin and then a length of bacon to wrap around outer edge.
Place the bacon in the oven for 10-15minutes until it starts to go crispy.
Whilst the bacon is cooking, peel and mash the avocados in a bowl. Add the hot sauce, a squeeze of lemon juice and a good pinch of salt and pepper. Combine well.
Remove the bacon from the oven (keep the oven on). Using a teaspoon, add the mashed avocado to the bacon rings. The bacon will have shrunk slightly, but try to fill the centre of the bacon. Make a well using the back of the spoon in the middle of each mould for the egg to sit in.
Crack an egg into the centre of each muffin mould. Place the tin back n the oven for 10 minutes until the eggs are cooked
Once the eggs are baked, remove from the oven and let them cool slightly. Run a knife around the edge of each cup and lift out with a spoon.

Notes
If you are using these for meal prep, let the cups completely cool, then pop in the fridge. Reheat them at 180ºc / 360ºf for 10 minutes.
Nutritional value based on 1 of 6 servings

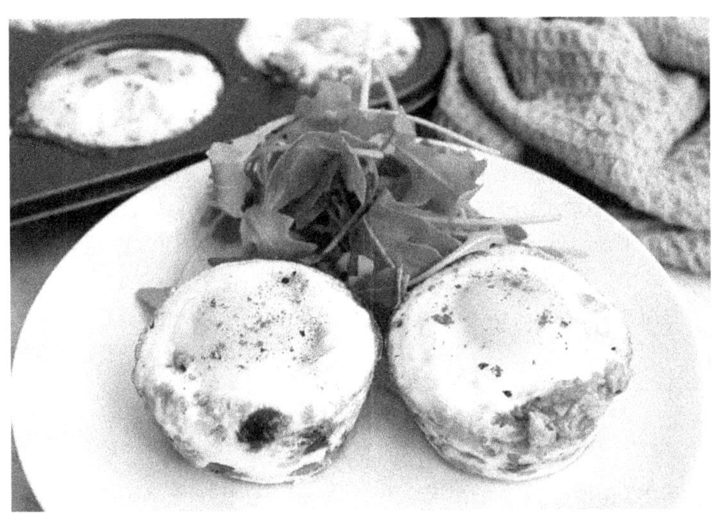

LUNCH

Creamy cauliflower soup with bacon and cheddar.

INGREDIENTS

1/2 pound sliced bacon, cut into 1/2-inch pieces
1 medium onion, finely chopped (about 1 1/2 cups)
6 scallions, white and pale green parts only, thinly sliced
4 medium cloves garlic, thinly sliced
1 quart homemade or store-bought low-sodium chicken stock,
plus more as needed
2 bay leaves
1 cup half-and-half or heavy cream
1 head cauliflower, cut into florets
Kosher salt and freshly ground black pepper

INSTRUCTION

Heat bacon in a large Dutch oven over medium-high heat, stirring constantly until bacon is completely crisp. Remove from Dutch oven with a slotted spoon and set aside, leaving fat in Dutch oven.

Add onions, half of scallions, and garlic, and cook, stirring constantly and scraping up browned bits from the bottom of the pan until onion is softened, about 5 minutes.

Add chicken stock, bay leaves, half-and-half (or cream), and cauliflower. Season to taste with salt and pepper. Cover and cook until cauliflower is completely tender, about 30 minutes.

Working in batches, blend soup until completely smooth (if you don't have a very powerful blender, remove the bay leaf before blending. If an extra-smooth soup is desired, pass the soup through a fine-mesh strainer after blending); if soup is too thick, whisk in additional hot chicken stock, 1/2 cup at a time, until you've reached the desired consistency. Season to taste with salt and pepper and serve sprinkled with crisp bacon pieces and remaining scallions.

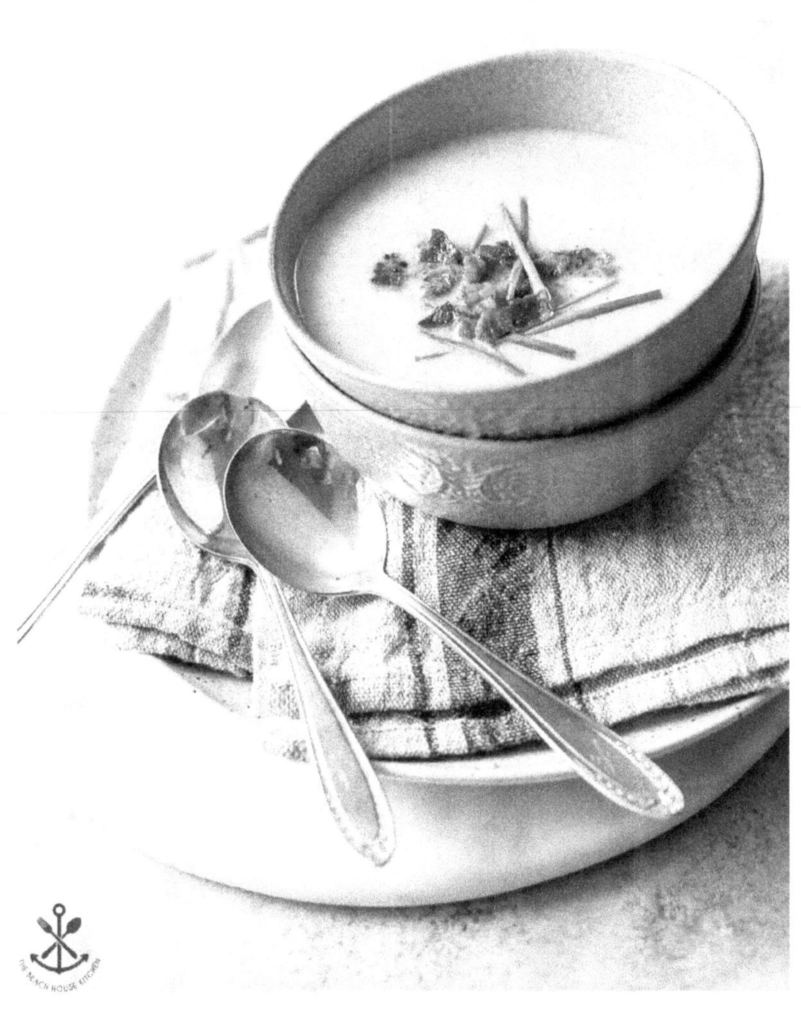

DINNER

Spinach and bacon salad with a creamy dressing

INGREDIENTS

Salad

10 -12 ounces fresh spinach, washed and torn into bit-size
pieces (I use the pre-packaged baby spinach)

1/4 cup minced red onion

Dressing

6 slices bacon, chopped

1/4 cup cider vinegar

1/4 cup Splenda granular (or sugar if desired)

1/4 cup mayonnaise

1/2 teaspoon salt

1/8 teaspoon pepper

Garnish

2 hard-boiled eggs, chopped

1 hard-boiled egg, sliced

INSTRUCTION

Place prepared spinach in a large bowl. Add onion.
Refrigerate, tightly covered.

Fry chopped bacon until crisp; remove to paper towel and set
aside.

Allow bacon drippings to cool for 5 minutes or so (until it is no
longer sizzling). In the frying pan, combine the drippings with
vinegar, Splenda (or sugar), mayonnaise, salt and pepper and
blend well.

You can now refrigerate all ingredients until just before
serving, storing the dressing in a covered microwaveable
container. OR you can use the dressing right out of the pan
and proceed to tossing the salad.

When ready to serve, microwave the dressing on HIGH for 30
to 45 seconds, or until mixture boils.

Toss the chopped egg with the spinach salad then pour the hot
dressing over greens mixture; toss again lightly.

Top with sliced egg and crumbled bacon.

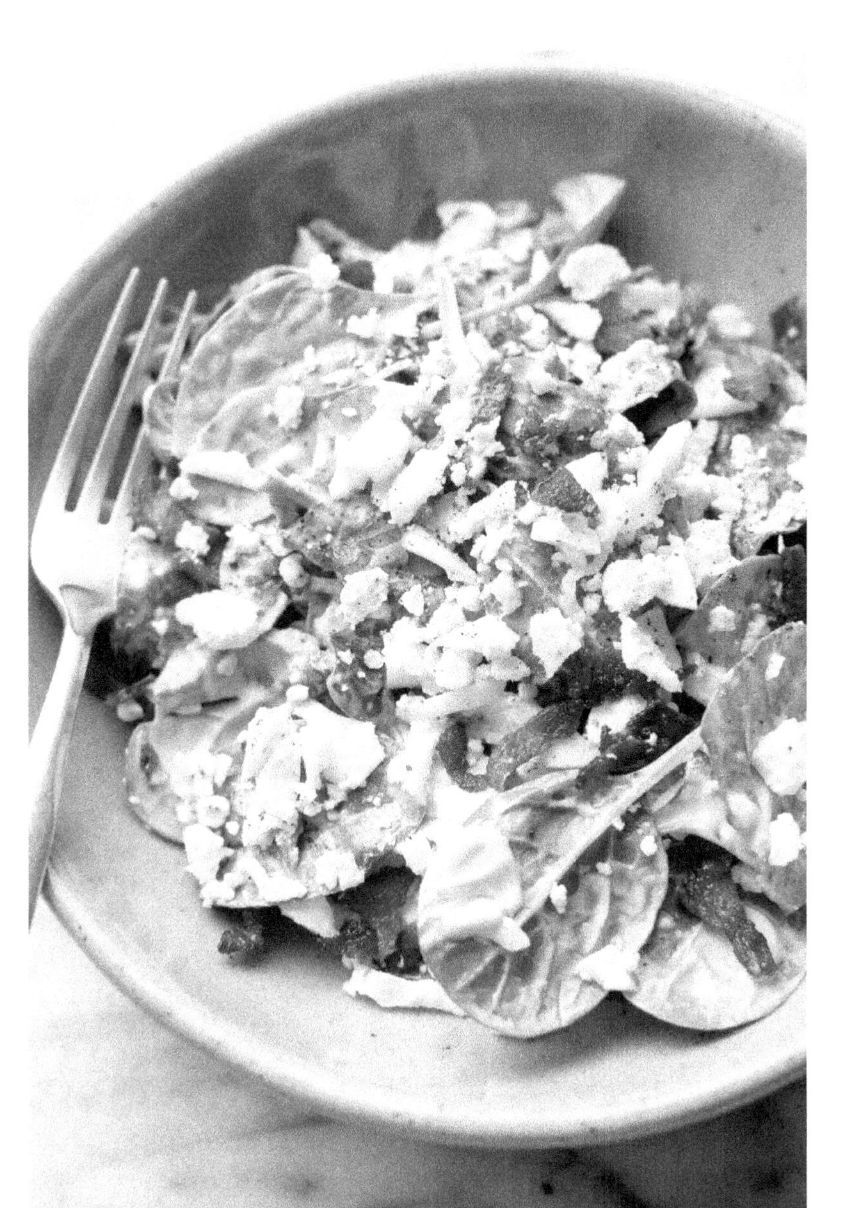

Day 15

Breakfast

Coconut flour waffles with whipped cream and strawberries.

Lunch

Broccoli and cheddar-stuffed portobello mushrooms.

Dinner

Shrimp scampi with zucchini noodles.

BREAKFAST

Coconut flour waffles with whipped cream and strawberries.

INGREDIENTS

2 tablespoon coconut flour
2 tablespoon coconut milk I used full fat canned coconut milk
2 tablespoon finely shredded coconut
1.5 tablespoon Joy Filled Eats Sweetener (or see alternatives in recipe notes)
2 tablespoon almond milk
1 egg
½ teaspoon vanilla
½ teaspoon baking powder
Ingredients for the sauce:
4 frozen strawberries

INSTRUCTION

Heat up your waffle iron.

Combine all the waffle ingredients and mix until smooth.

Grease waffle iron with cooking spray or coconut oil. Pour on batter (it will be thick).

Cook until golden. Put on a plate.

Make the sauce. Microwave the strawberries in a small bowl for about 90 seconds until thawed and warmed. Using kitchen shears cut up right in the bowl.

Dump the strawberry sauce on your waffle. Enjoy!

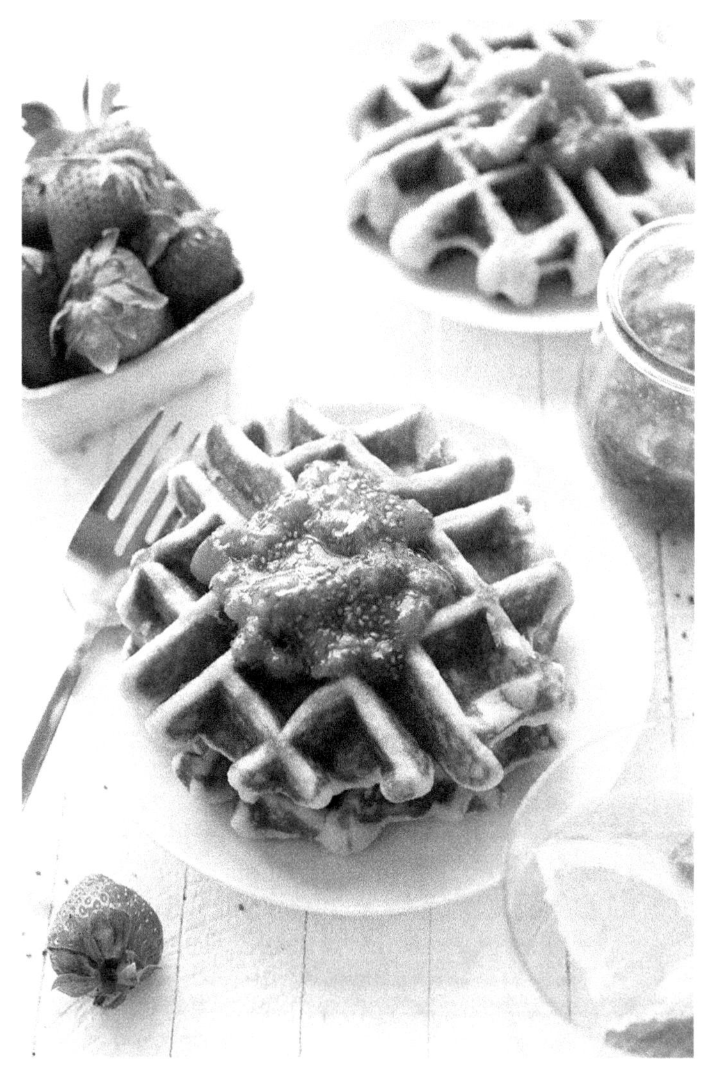

LUNCH

Broccoli and cheddar-stuffed portobello mushrooms.

INGREDIENTS

6 large portabello mushroom caps
olive oil cooking spray or olive oil in a mister
10 oz fresh broccoli florets
1 cup fresh bread crumbs made from day-old bread
2 Tbsp fresh Italian parsley chopped
1 Tbsp fresh thyme leaves chopped
1 egg lightly beaten
½ + 1/4 t kosher salt divided
pinch fresh cracked pepper
2 tsp unsalted butter
2 tsp all-purpose flour
1 cup milk not skim
1 cup shredded sharp cheddar cheese
1 tsp country-style Dijon mustard

INSTRUCTION

Heat oven to 400F. Bring a large pot of water to a boil.
Prepare the mushrooms: wipe off any dirt with a lightly damp
paper towel. Remove the stems and discard (these can be saved,
diced, and added to the stuffing, but mine were tough so I didn't
save them). Using a spoon, gently scrape off the gills on the
underside of the mushroom caps. Spray both sides with olive oil
and place upside down on a bake sheet.
Blanch the broccoli in the boiling water 2 minutes. Transfer to a ice
bath to stop the cooking. Drain. Chop finely (this can be
accomplished easily with a mini chopper or by pulsing in a food
processor).
In a large bowl, combine the chopped broccoli, bread crumbs,
parsley, thyme, egg, 1/2 t salt, and pepper. Distribute the stuffing
into the mushrooms. Bake at 400F for 15 minutes or until
mushrooms are cooked through and juicy and the stuffing is lightly
browned.
While the mushrooms are cooking, prepare the cheese sauce. In a
medium saucepan over medium-high heat, whisk the butter and
flour until smooth and bubbly.

Cook an additional minute to cook the flour. Whisking constantly, slowly add in the milk. Cook, stirring constantly, until thickened enough to coat the back of a wooden spoon. Remove from the heat and whisk in the cheese, Dijon, and 1/4 t salt until smooth. Serve the stuffed mushrooms with sauce drizzled over. Yield: 3 servings as a main course; 6 as a side.

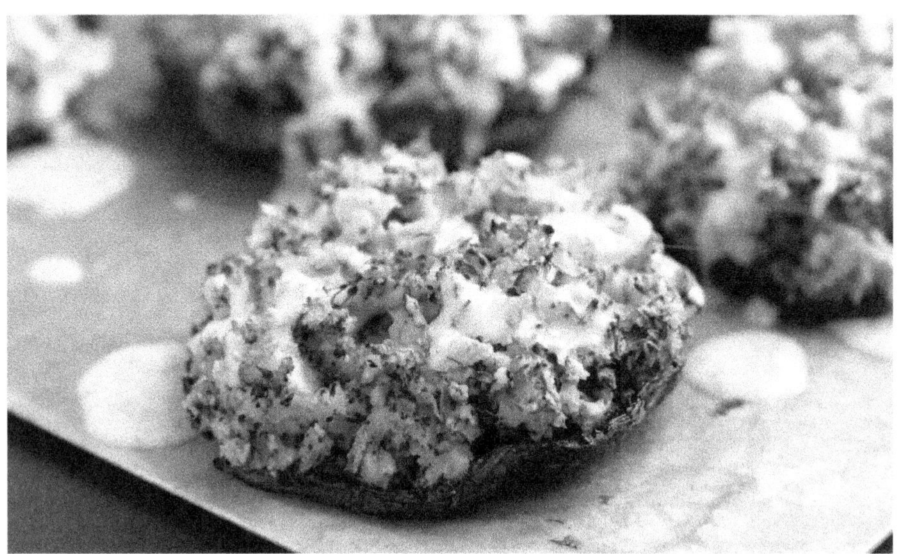

DINNER

Shrimp scampi with zucchini noodles.

INGREDIENTS

1 tablespoon unsalted butter
1 tablespoon olive oil
1 shallot finely chopped
4 cloves garlic minced (about 1 1/2 tablespoons)
1 pound large raw shrimp peeled and deveined with tails on
(fresh or frozen and thawed)
1 teaspoon kosher salt
1/2 teaspoon red pepper flakes
1/4 teaspoon black pepper
1/4 cup low-sodium chicken broth or white wine
Zest of 1/2 lemon
1/4 cup freshly squeezed lemon juice
1 1/2 pounds zucchini noodles from about 4 medium zucchini
1/4 cup chopped fresh parsley leaves
2 tablespoons freshly grated Parmesan

INSTRUCTION

Heat the butter and olive oil in a large skillet over medium-low heat. Add the shallot and cook until beginning to soften, about 3 minutes. Add the garlic and cook 30 seconds. Add the shrimp, salt, red pepper flakes, and black pepper. Sauté for 3 minutes, until the shrimp are beginning to cook but are still somewhat translucent.
Add the chicken broth, lemon zest, and lemon juice. Bring to a boil and cook for 1 minute, just until the shrimp are completely opaque and cooked through. Stir in the zucchini noodles and parsley. Toss the noodles with the shrimp so that they are coated with the garlic-lemon sauce and heat just until warmed through. (Do not overcook or the zucchini noodles will become mushy.) Sprinkle with parsley and Parmesan. Serve warm.

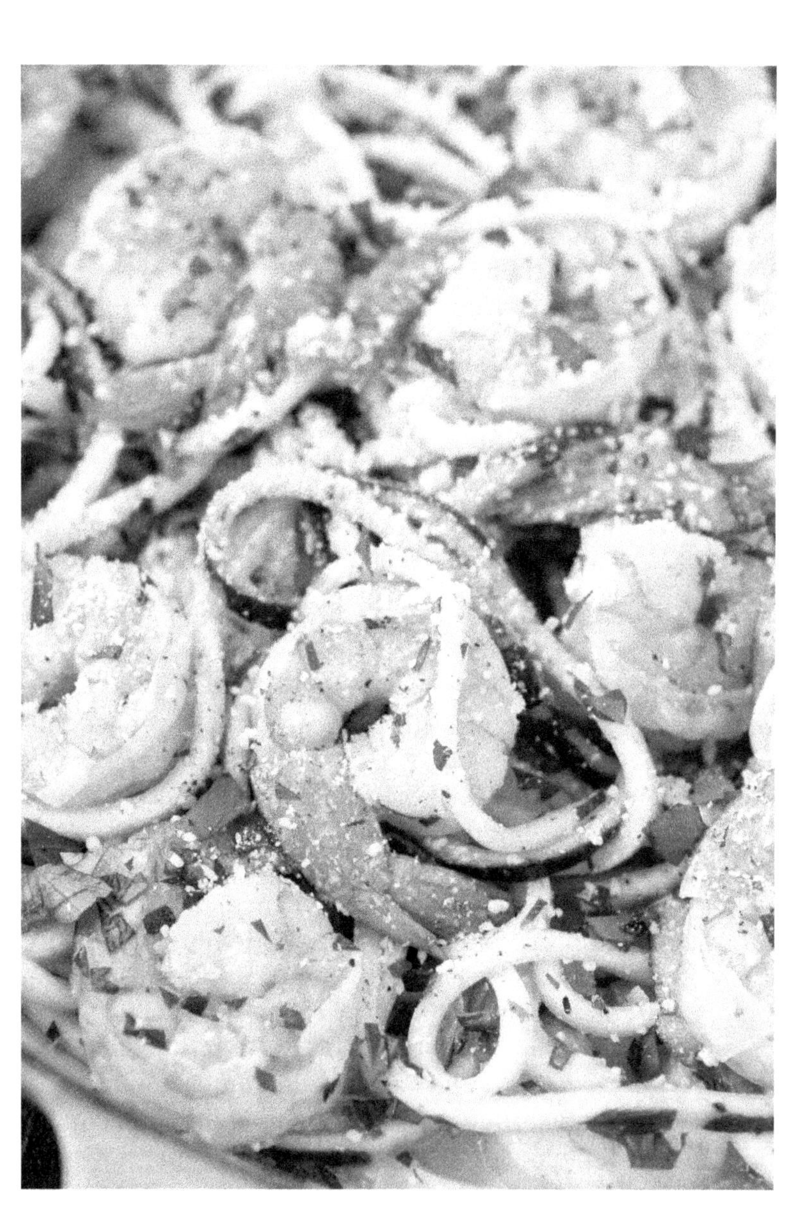

Day 16

Breakfast

Breakfast salad with mixed greens, avocado, and poached eggs.

Lunch

Greek chicken souvlaki with a side of Greek salad.

Dinner

Grilled chicken Caesar salad with homemade dressing.

BREAKFAST

Breakfast salad with mixed greens, avocado, and poached eggs.

INGREDIENTS

2 large eggs
4 cups lettuce (or greens of choice)
7 grape tomatoes
1 medium avocado
1/2 cup cooked quinoa
2 Tbsp chopped walnuts
salt/pepper (to taste)

INSTRUCTION

Bring a small pot of water to a boil.

Give the water a swirl, then place the egg poachers in the pot.

Pour the eggs into the poachers and let cook for 2-4 minutes.

Create the salads by layering the lettuce, tomatoes, avocado, cooked quinoa, and walnuts.

Add the poached eggs and top with salt/pepper to taste.

Enjoy!

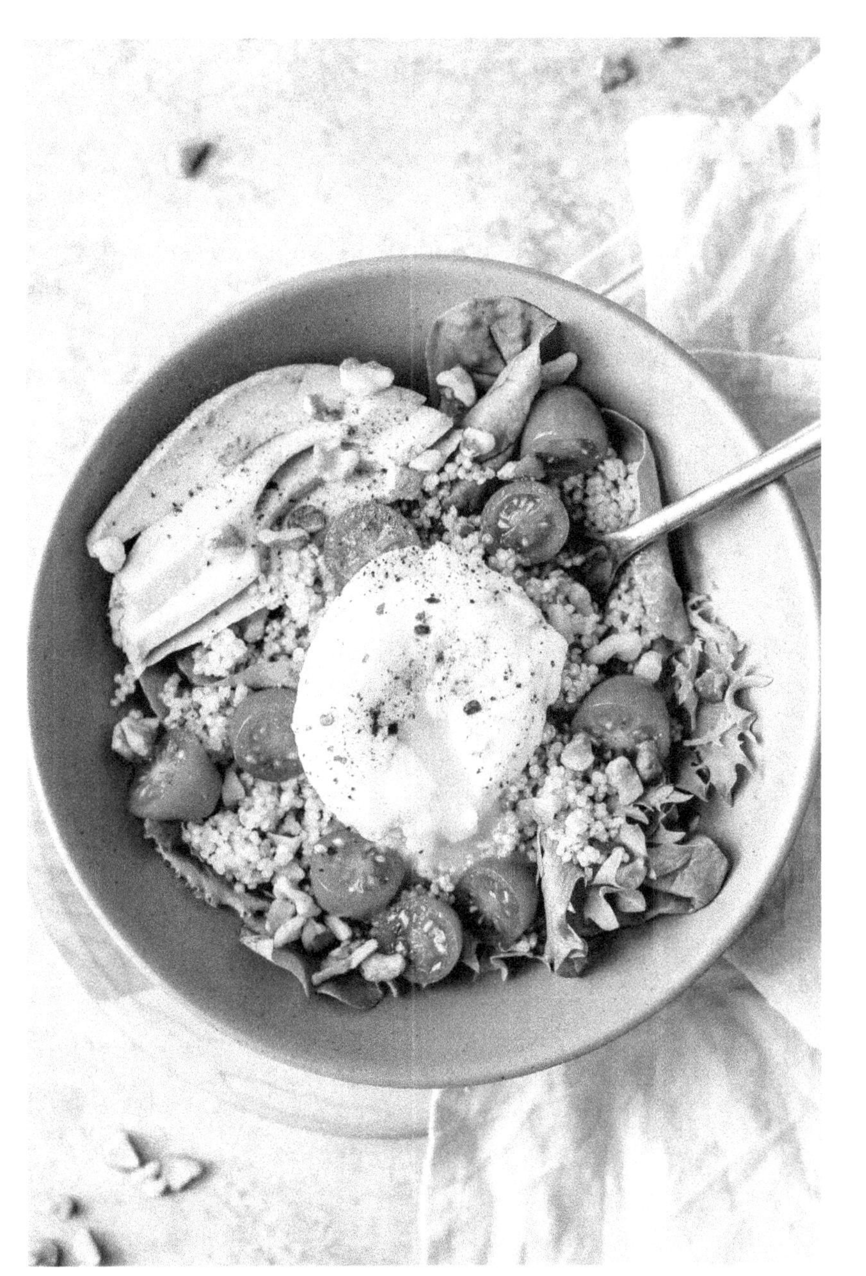

LUNCH

Greek chicken souvlaki with a side of Greek salad.

INGREDIENTS

For the Chicken:

5 tablespoons fresh juice from about 3 lemons
4 tablespoons red wine vinegar
4 tablespoons olive oil
2 tablespoons chopped fresh oregano leaves
2 teaspoons kosher salt
1/2 teaspoon ground black pepper
2 pounds skinless boneless chicken breast, trimmed of excess fat
and cut into 1-inch pieces
4 medium cloves garlic, grated (about 4 teaspoons)
For the Tzatziki Sauce:

1 medium cucumber, peeled, seeded, cut into 1/4-inch cubes (see
notes)
1/2 teaspoon salt
1 medium clove garlic, grated (about 1 teaspoon)
1 cup Greek yogurt (see notes)
1 tablespoon chopped fresh dill
For the Salad:

2 tablespoons olive oil
6 small tomatoes, cut into wedges
2 small red onions, sliced thin
1 medium cucumber, seeded and sliced into thin half moons
3/4 cup pitted Kalamata olives
6 ounces crumbled feta
1/4 cup chopped parsley
6 pitas

INSTRUCTION

In a medium bowl, whisk lemon juice, vinegar, olive oil, oregano, salt, and black pepper. Place chicken cubes in a separate medium bowl. Mix in grated garlic and 7 tablespoons of dressing. Toss chicken to coat evenly, cover, and refrigerate to marinate for about 2 hours, tossing occasionally. Set remaining dressing aside for salad.In a medium bowl, whisk lemon juice, vinegar, olive oil, oregano, salt, and black pepper. Place chicken cubes in a separate medium bowl. Mix in grated garlic and 7 tablespoons of dressing. Toss chicken to coat evenly, cover, and refrigerate to marinate for about 2 hours, tossing occasionally. Set remaining dressing aside for salad.

While the chicken marinates, make the tzatziki sauce: Place cubed cucumbers in a strainer set over a bowl. Toss with 1/2 teaspoon salt and let sit to drain, about 30 minutes. Gently pat cucumbers dry with paper towel, place in small bowl, and mix with garlic, yogurt, and dill. Season to taste with salt. Refrigerate until ready to serve.

Skewer chicken pieces on 8 to 12 skewers. Discard used marinade. Heat grill or grill pan over medium-high heat. Place chicken skewers on grill (or cook in batches on grill pan) until well browned and internal temperature registers 155°F (68°C) on an instant-read thermometer, turning evenly to cook on all sides, about 5 minutes total. (Adjust temperature of grill if necessary.) Remove chicken to a serving platter and let rest 3 minutes. Meanwhile, briefly grill pitas and keep warm.

Just before serving, prepare the salad: Whisk olive oil into reserved chicken marinade. Add tomatoes, onions, cucumber, olives, feta, and parsley. Season with salt and pepper.

Serve skewers with salad, pita, and tzatziki sauce. Remove chicken from skewers to stuff into pitas with sauce and salad.

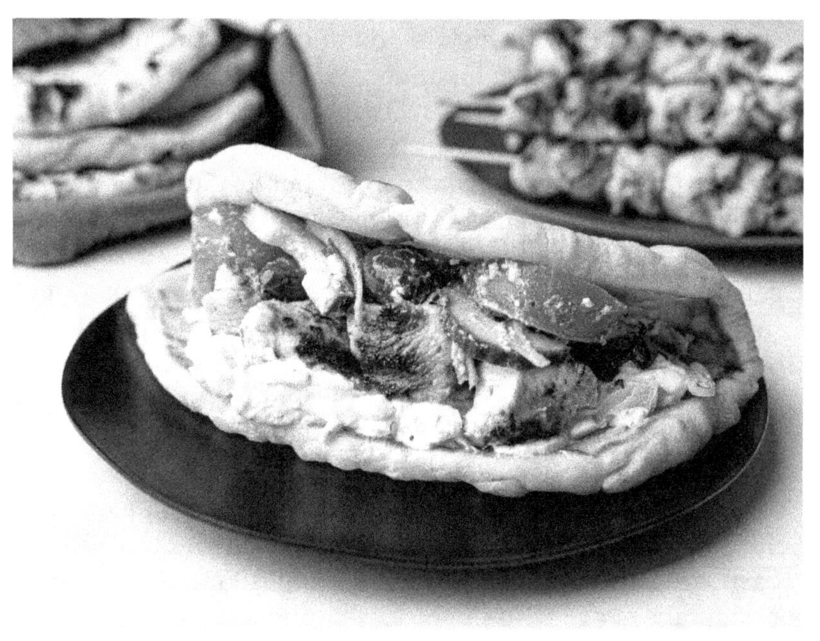

DINNER

Grilled chicken Caesar salad with homemade dressing.

INGREDIENTS

Chicken Marinade
1/2 of a lemon, juiced
1 tablespoon olive oil
2 tablespoons dijon mustard
1 clove of garlic, mined
1 tablespoon fresh rosemary, minced
3/4 teaspoon kosher salt
Fresh ground black pepper to taste
1 pound boneless skinless chicken breasts

Salad
2 romaine hearts, halved lengthwise
4 slices whole wheat bread, a crusty artisan type is best
2 tablespoons grated parmesan cheese
Kosher salt and fresh ground black pepper

Caesar Dressing
1/2 cup plain non-fat Greek yogurt
1/2 of a lemon, juiced
2 teaspoons olive oil
2 teaspoons red wine vinegar
2 teaspoons worchestershire
2 teaspoons dijon mustard
1 teaspoon anchovy paste
1/4 teaspoon granulated garlic
1/4 cup shredded parmesan cheese
Kosher salt and fresh ground black pepper to taste

INSTRUCTION

Chicken Marinade

In a small bowl whisk together the ingredients for the marinade. Season the chicken with salt and pepper then place it in a freezer bag.
Pour the marinade over the chicken, seal the bag, then massage it into the chicken with your hands. Refrigerate for at least an hour.
Caesar Dressing

add all of the ingredients to a bowl and whisk together until combined. Cover and refrigerate until ready to serve.
Salad

Preheat grill to medium-high heat and brush the grill grates with oil.
Place the marinated chicken onto the grill and cook for 4-6 minutes depending on the thickness, then flip over and cook another 4-6 minutes or until cooked through (165 degrees F.).
Remove the chicken from the grill and let it rest while you grill the romaine hearts and bread.
Drizzle olive oil on the romaine hearts and slices of bread and season them with kosher salt and freshly ground black pepper.
Place the romaine hearts cut side down on the grill and cook them for approximately 2-3 minutes or until they have nice grill marks.
Grill the bread at the same time as the lettuce for approximately 1 minute per side. Once grilled, cut the bread into bite sized cubes.
Place the grilled romaine hearts cut side up on a serving platter and top them with slices of the grilled chicken, cubes of the grilled bread, Caesar dressing, shredded parmesan cheese and season with kosher salt and freshly ground black pepper.

Serve immediately.

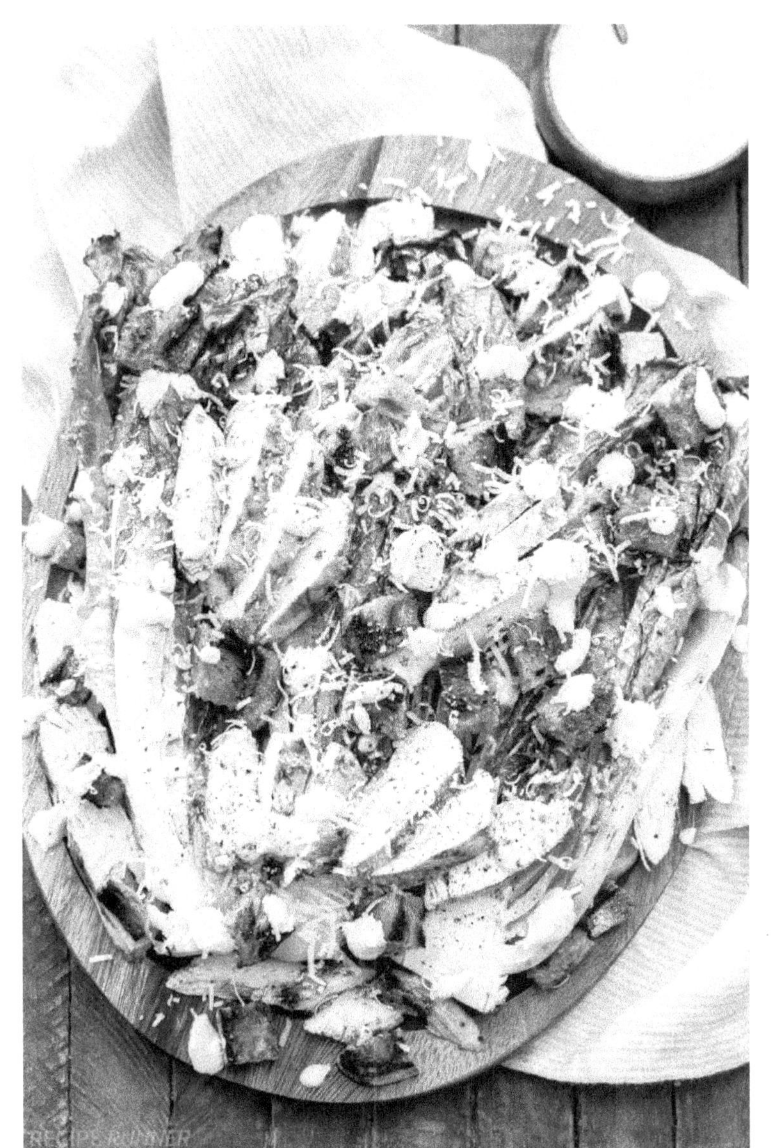

Day 17

Breakfast

Cauliflower hash browns with eggs and salsa.

Lunch

Chicken and vegetable stir-fry with soy sauce.

Dinner

Beef and broccoli stir-fry with sesame seeds.

BREAKFAST

Cauliflower hash browns with eggs and salsa.

INGREDIENTS

750 g Cauliflower Hash Browns
200 ml Double Cream
250 g Red Leicester
30 g Pickled Jalapeños
2 Tomatoes
1 Red Onion
1 Red Chilli
15 g Coriander
2 Limes
4 Egg

INSTRUCTION

Preheat the oven to 200°C.
Lay the hash browns onto a tray lined with parchment paper.
Chuck the hash browns into the oven and cook until crispy and golden. This will take roughly 12-13 mins.
Meanwhile, add the double cream to a small saucepan and gently warm. Coarsely grate the red Leicester and stir into the cream to gently melt. Roughly chop the jalapeños and stir through the cheesy sauce. Add a splash of the pickle brine for extra tang if you fancy.
Finely chop the tomatoes, red onion and red chilli. Chuck them into a mixing bowl and stir together with a big pinch of salt. Roughly chop the coriander and stir through the mix with the juice of one lime.
Fry the eggs until crispy and cut the remaining lime into wedges.
Layer up your hash browns, salsa, cheese sauce, and top with eggs and lime wedges.

Get stuck in.

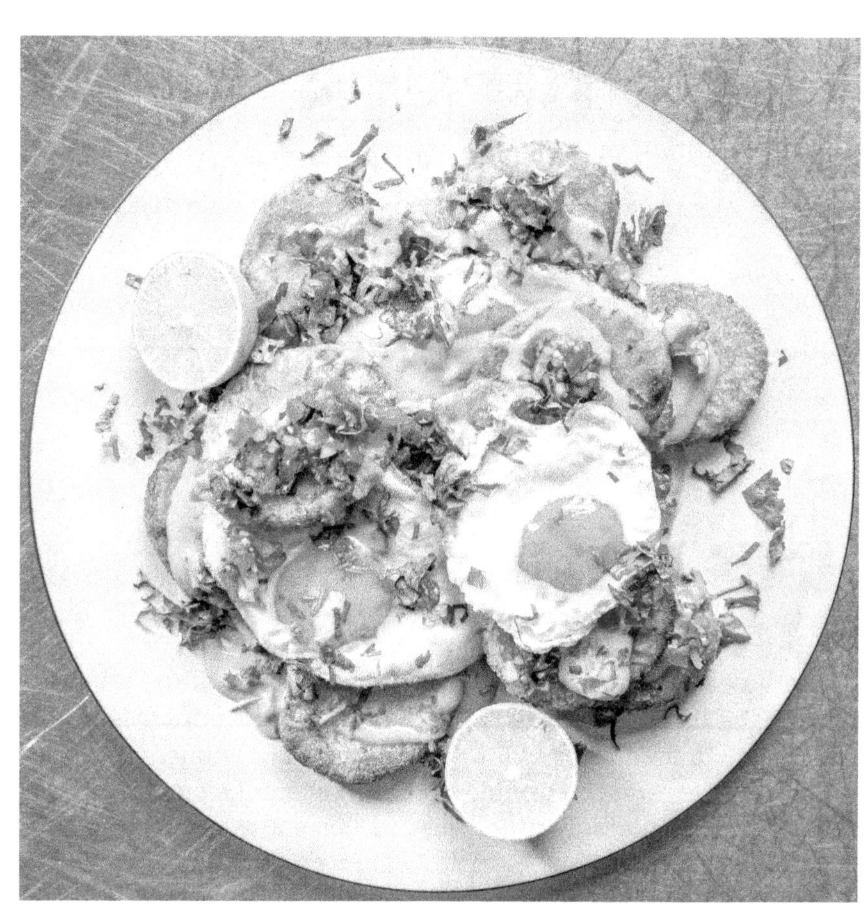

LUNCH

Chicken and vegetable stir-fry with soy sauce.

INGREDIENTS

1 lb boneless, skinless chicken breast cut into 1 inch cubes
salt and pepper to taste
2 tbsp olive oil divided
2 cups broccoli florets
1/2 yellow bell pepper cut into 1 inch pieces
1/2 red bell pepper cut into 1 inch pieces
1/2 cup baby carrots sliced
2 tsp minced ginger
2 garlic cloves minced
Stir Fry Sauce
1 tbsp corn starch
2 tbsp cold water
1/4 cup low sodium chicken broth
3 tbsp low sodium soy sauce
1/4 cup honey
1 tbsp toasted sesame oil
1/2 tsp crushed red pepper flakes

INSTRUCTION

Stir Fry Sauce
In a medium size bowl, whisk together corn starch and water.
Add remaining ingredients (chicken broth, soy sauce, honey,
and toasted sesame oil, red pepper flakes) and whisk to
combine. Set aside
Add one tablespoon of olive oil to a large skillet or wok and heat
over medium high heat
Add chicken (in batches if necessary) and season with salt and
pepper. Cook for 3 to 5 minutes or until cooked through.
Remove from skillet
Reduce heat to medium and add remaining tablespoon of oil to
the skillet
Add broccoli, bell pepper, and carrots and cook, stirring
occasionally, just until crisp tender. Add ginger and garlic and
cook for an additional minute.....nute.

Add chicken back into the skillet and stir to combine.
Whisk stir fry sauce and pour over chicken and vegetables
and stir gently to combine.
Bring to a boil, stirring occasionally, and let boil for one
minute.
Serve with rice and/or chow mein if desired.

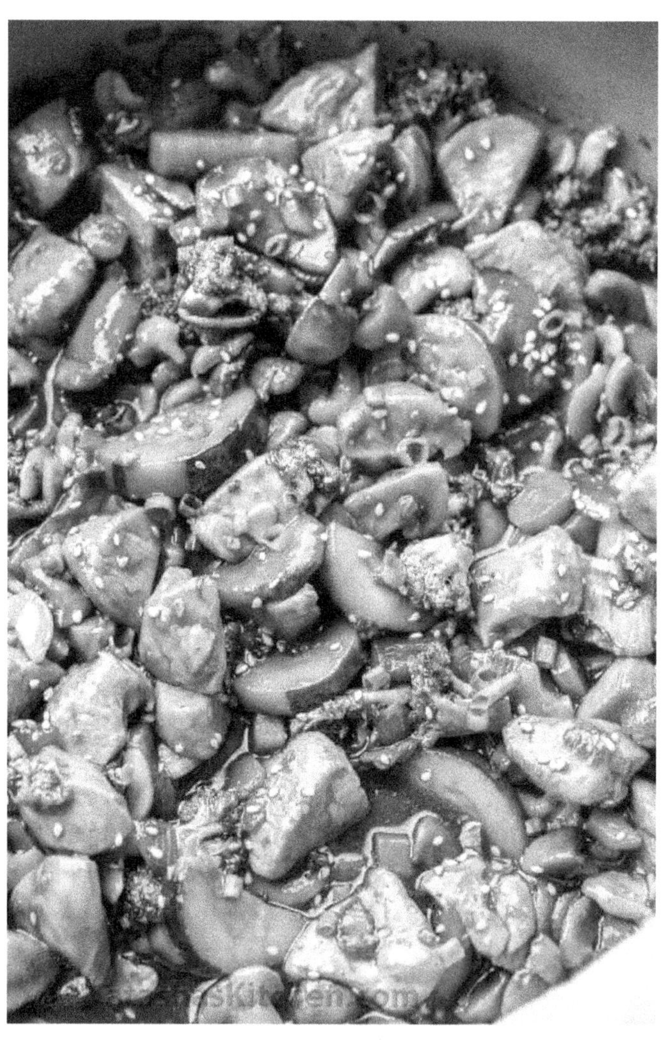

DINNER

Beef and broccoli stir-fry with sesame seeds.

INGREDIENTS

The Basics:
1 lb. beef flank steak, thinly sliced
1 head broccoli, cut into florets
2 tablespoons vegetable oil
3 cloves garlic, thinly sliced or minced
one 1-inch knob fresh peeled ginger, grated or sliced
1.5 cups of uncooked white rice or brown rice, (or a bag of cauliflower rice)
thinly sliced green onions for serving
The Sauce:
1/4 cup low sodium soy sauce
1/4 cup water
1/3 cup brown sugar (sub coconut sugar)
1 tablespoon sambal oelek
1 tablespoon rice vinegar (sub white vinegar)
1 tablespoon sesame oil
1 tablespoon cornstarch

INSTRUCTION

Beef Prep: Freeze beef for 30 minutes – 1 hour for easier slicing. Slice against the grain, into very thin strips. Toss the beef strips with a generous pinch of coarse salt and let it rest while you prep everything else. (All of this is optional but recommended for flavor and texture.)

Sauce: Whisk the sauce ingredients together.

Rice: Cook your rice according to package directions.

Stir Fry Time: Heat a large heavy skillet over medium heat. Add a swish of oil. Working in batches, add the beef in a single layer. Let rest, undisturbed, for a minute or two to achieve a nice browning on the meat. Flip each piece over and cook until browned and yummy. Remove beef from pan.

Broccoli: Add a swish of oil to the same pan. Add the broccoli; stir fry for 2-3 minutes, until bright green. (Sometimes I add a splash of water to steam it a little bit.) Remove broccoli from pan.

Finally: Turn the heat down and let the pan cool a bit. Add one last swish of oil. Add the ginger and garlic; sauté for 1-2 minutes. Add the sauce; stir until a thickened and sticky sauce forms. Add beef and broccoli back in. Toss gently to coat.
YUM! Serve with rice, thinly sliced green onions, and sesame seeds.

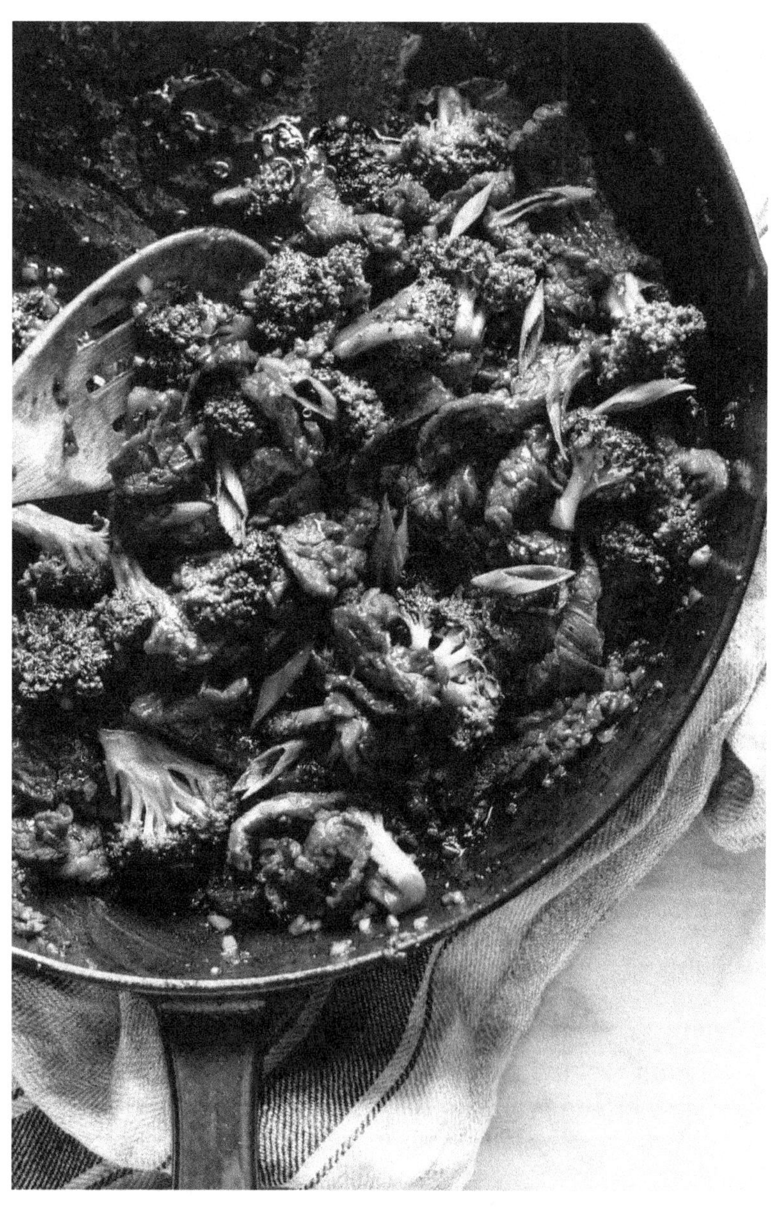

Day 18

Breakfast

Zucchini and cheese mini fritters.

Lunch

Avocado and bacon-stuffed cherry tomatoes.

Dinner

Eggplant and mozzarella stacks with tomato and basil

BREAKFAST

Zucchini and cheese mini fritters.

INGREDIENTS

1½ cups shredded zucchini skin left on
¾ cup finely crushed Ritz crackers or other similar cracker about
½ of a sleeve
½ cup shredded cheddar cheese
1 egg
3 tablespoons grated yellow onion
½ teaspoon seasoning salt blend or ¼ 1/4 teaspoon each of salt
and pepper
2 tablespoons canola, olive, or vegetable oil for frying

INSTRUCTION

Shred enough zucchini for 1 and 1/2 cups. Put the zucchini shreds in a colander and press down with a paper towel. The liquid should drain. (Blot out as much moisture as possible in order to get crispy zucchini fritters.)
Transfer the zucchini shreds to a medium-sized mixing bowl. Add all other ingredients and stir to combine.
Let the mixture rest for 10 minutes to allow the crackers to soften and the mixture ingredients to bind together.
Heat the oil in a skillet or electric frying pan over medium heat for about 3 minutes.
While the oil is heating, shape the cheesy zucchini fritter mixture into 2 or 3 inch balls. Flatten slightly with your hand to form a zucchini patty or cake shape. Note: If you make the fritters into 1 inch balls, then flatten, you could call them cheesy zucchini bites.
While the oil is heating, shape the cheesy zucchini fritter mixture into 2 or 3 inch balls. Flatten slightly with your hand to form a zucchini patty or cake shape. Note: If you make the fritters into 1 inch balls, then flatten, you could call them cheesy zucchini bites.
When the time is up, remove the zucchini fritters from the pan and drain on a plate covered with paper towels.

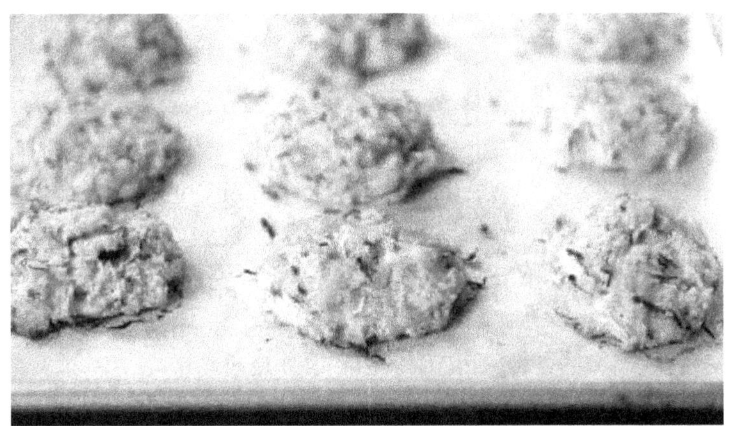

LUNCH

Avocado and bacon-stuffed cherry tomatoes.

INGREDIENTS

1 pint cherry tomatoes
1 large avocado, peeled and mashed
4 teaspoons lemon juice
1 tablespoon finely chopped onion
1 clove garlic, minced
1/2 cup finely shredded swiss cheese
1/4 teaspoon seasoning salt
6 slices bacon, cooked and finely crumbled or 6 slices bottled
bacon bits (optional)

INSTRUCTION

Remove the tops from the tomatoes.

Scoop out and discard the seeds.

Drain cut-side down on paper towels.

In a small bowl beat together the avocado through seasoned
salt until smooth.

Stuff the avocado mixture into the tomatoes.

Serve sprinkled w/ bacon bits.

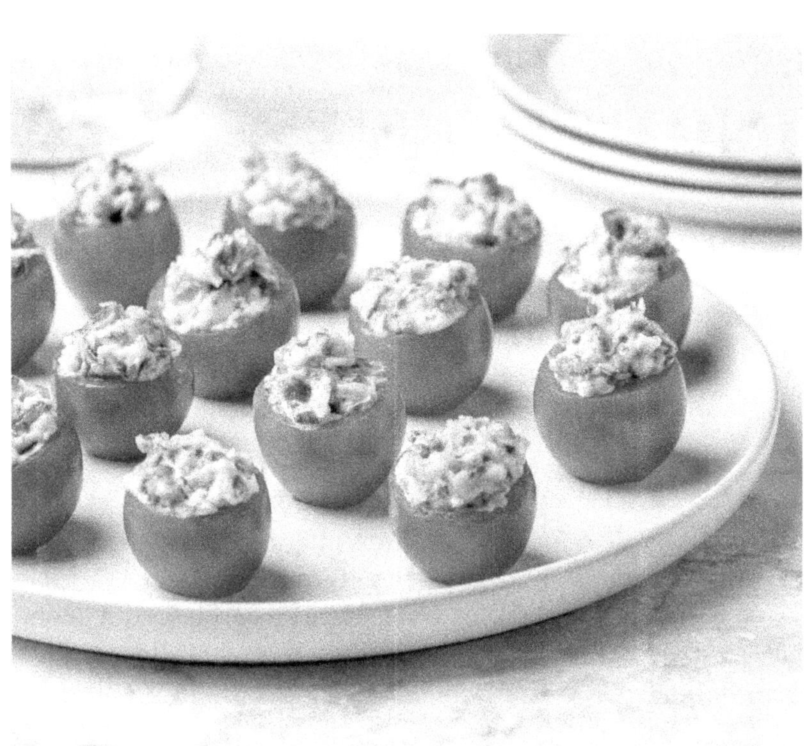

DINNER

Eggplant and mozzarella stacks with tomato and basil.

INGREDIENTS

2 eggplants (nicely round, not slender)
4 teaspoons olive oil (or more)
2 large ripe tomatoes
8 slices mozzarella cheese (pre-spiced is fine)
finely chopped herbs (like basil, oreganum, thyme)
salt and black pepper
4 tablespoons vinaigrette dressing (if making this a salad)

INSTRUCTION

Heat oven to 350 deg F/180 deg Celsius.
From each eggplant/aubergine, slice 6 rounds, about 1/3" thick.
Discard the thinner ends. You now have 12 rounds. Put a sheet of
nonstick baking paper on a cookie tin. Arrange the slices in a
single layer, and drizzle each with a little olive oil.
Bake for about 15 minutes, or until the slices are soft -- do not
burn. Cool and keep.
To assemble, slice each tomato into 4 even slices, discarding the
ends, so you have 8 tomato slices.
Chop your herbs of choice finely, or use dried herbs if fresh herbs
are not available.
Starting with an eggplant slice, stack each of 4 stacks as follows:
eggplant, tomato, mozzarella, eggplant again, tomato slice,
eggplant, mozzarella slice.
SEASON each layer lightly as you go, with just tiny pinches of salt,
and a sprinkle of herbs and black pepper.
You will have 4 stacks, serving 2 - 4 people.
As a warm side dish: heat gently in a warm oven (under cooking
point of 212 deg F) until the tomato slices are warm and the
mozzarella melts. Delicious with fried chicken pieces/.
As a salad: drizzle with a tangy French vinaigrette and serve with
toasted bruschetta slices.

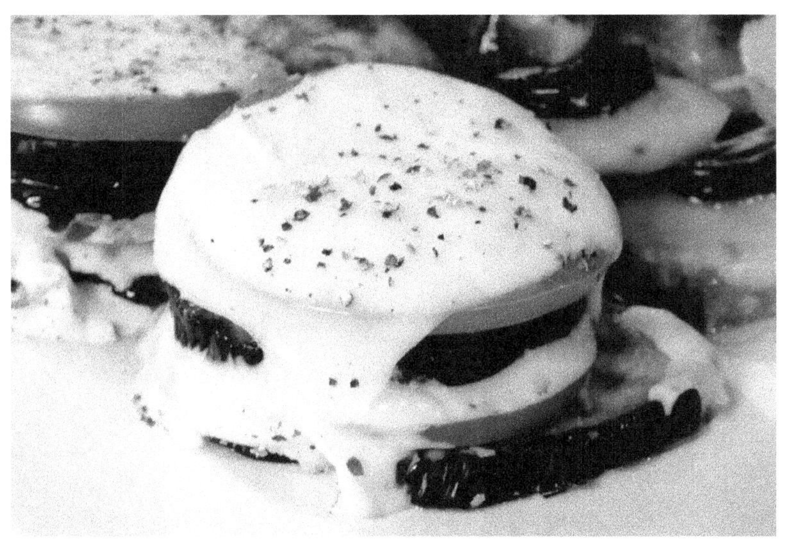

Day 19

Breakfast

Sausage and
vegetable skillet.

Lunch

Mediterranean
quinoa bowl with
olives and feta.

Dinner

Salmon and
avocado nori rolls

BREAKFAST

Sausage and vegetable skillet.

INGREDIENTS

1 Tbsp cooking oil
1 lb. Italian sausage
1/2 lb. frozen cauliflower florets
1/2 lb. frozen peppers and onions
1/4 lb. frozen kale
½ tsp seasoning salt or seasoning blend (or to taste)

INSTRUCTION

Add the cooking oil and sausage to a skillet. Cook the sausage over medium heat until brown and crispy.

Add the cauliflower, peppers and onions, and kale to the skillet with the sausage. Continue to stir and cook until the vegetables are heated through.

Add a liberal amount (or to taste) of your favorite seasoning salt or seasoning blend and stir to combine.

Serve hot.

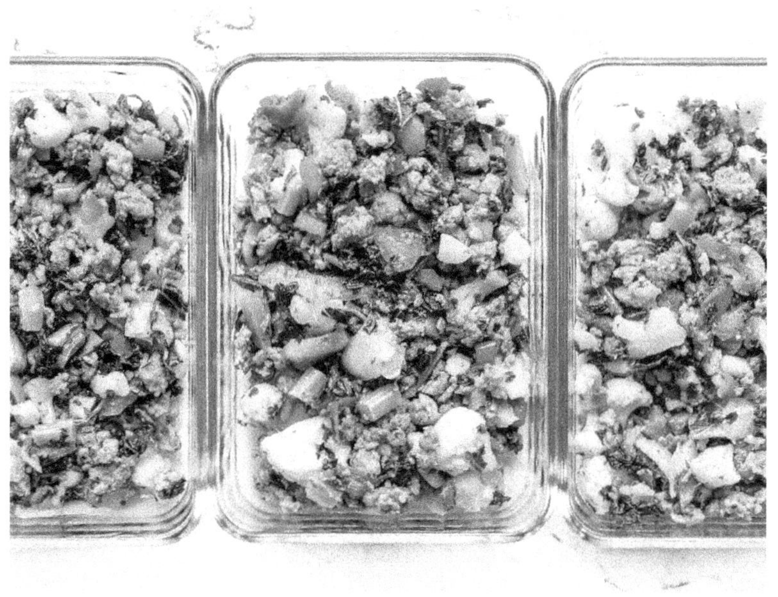

LUNCH

Mediterranean quinoa bowl with olives and feta.

INGREDIENTS

⅔ cup dry quinoa
1 ⅓ cup water
CHICKPEAS
1 15 oz can chickpeas, drained, rinsed and patted dry
1 teaspoon olive oil
1 teaspoon lemon juice
½ teaspoon oregano
½ teaspoon garlic powder
½ teaspoon salt
¼ teaspoon pepper
BOWL
4 cups baby spinach or arugula, loosely packed
1 cup cucumber, chopped
1 cup cherry tomatoes, chopped
½ cup red onion, chopped
½ cup feta cheese, crumbled
¼ cup kalamata olives
Lemon Vinaigrette
Hummus, for serving
Tzatziki Sauce, for drizzling
Fresh parsley, for serving

INSTRUCTION

Preheat oven to 400°F and line a baking sheet with parchment paper.

Rinse and drain quinoa, if desired. Add quinoa and water to a saucepan and bring to a boil. Reduce to a simmer, cover and cook for 15 minutes. Fluff with a fork and let cool for 5-10 minutes Add the chickpeas to a mixing bowl with oil and seasonings. Use your hands to coat the chickpeas well. Pour chickpeas onto a baking sheet. Bake for 20 minutes flipping halfway. Once cooked, set aside to cool.

If you haven't already, make the dressing and set aside.

To make the bowls, add about ½ cup cooked quinoa, 1 cup greens, ¼ cup cucumber, ¼ cup tomatoes, 2 Tablespoons onion, 2 Tablespoons feta cheese, 1 Tablespoon kalamata olives and scoop of hummus to 4 bowls. Divide chickpeas evenly and add to bowls then drizzle with tzatziki and dressing. Serve immediately.

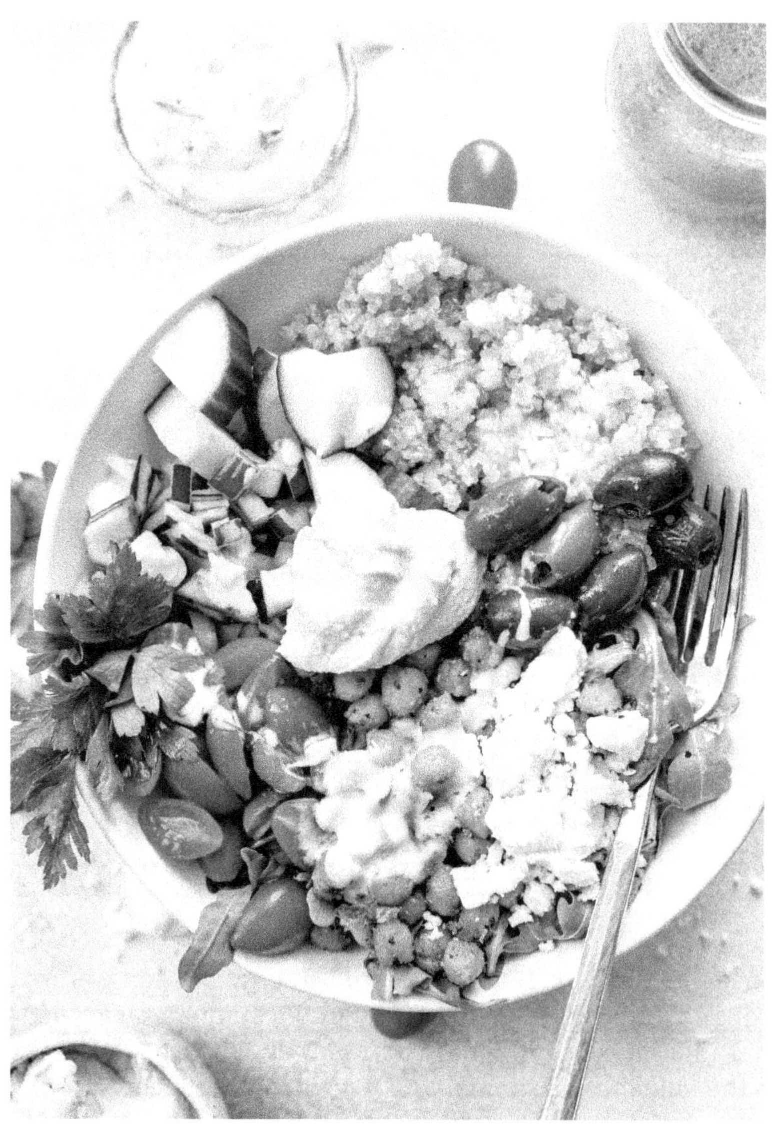

DINNER

Salmon and avocado nori rolls.

INGREDIENTS

1 1/2 cups rice, uncooked

Fresh salmon, sushi grade, sliced approximately 1/2″ square by 3-1/2″ long

1 avocado, sliced thinly lengthwise

4 green leaf lettuce leaves

3 sheets dried seaweed

3 Tbsp. Mizkan Seasoned Rice Vinegar

1 Tbsp. mayonnaise

½ tsp. chili oil or ¼ tsp red pepper flakes

White roasted sesame seeds for sprinkling on top of sushi roll, optional

INSTRUCTION

Cook sushi rice. Sprinkle Mizkan Seasoned Rice Vinegar over hot cooked rice. While mixing the rice and vinegar, cool rice quickly by fanning at the same time over the rice to make Sushi rice. Mix vinegar into rice in slicing motions after sprinkling sushi vinegar over the rice.

Spread prepared sushi rice thinly on a sheet of dried seaweed leaving approx. 1/2″ on both vertical edges. Makes enough sushi rice for 3 Salmon and Avocado rolls.

Spread a sheet of plastic wrap, large enough to line a seaweed sheet, on a cutting board, then lay the wrap gently down with the rice facing the plastic wrap.

Mix mayonnaise with chili oil or red pepper flakes well. Brush the mixture lightly on the seaweed. Lay each salmon slice, avocado slice, and a lettuce leaf on top of the seaweed sheet. Start rolling the rice into a log shape using plastic wrap as a guide to shape a firm rolled rice.

Separate the plastic wrap from the rice roll and sprinkle the top of the rolled rice with the roasted sesame seeds. Slice the finished salmon avocado roll into five to six slices with sharp knife and serve.

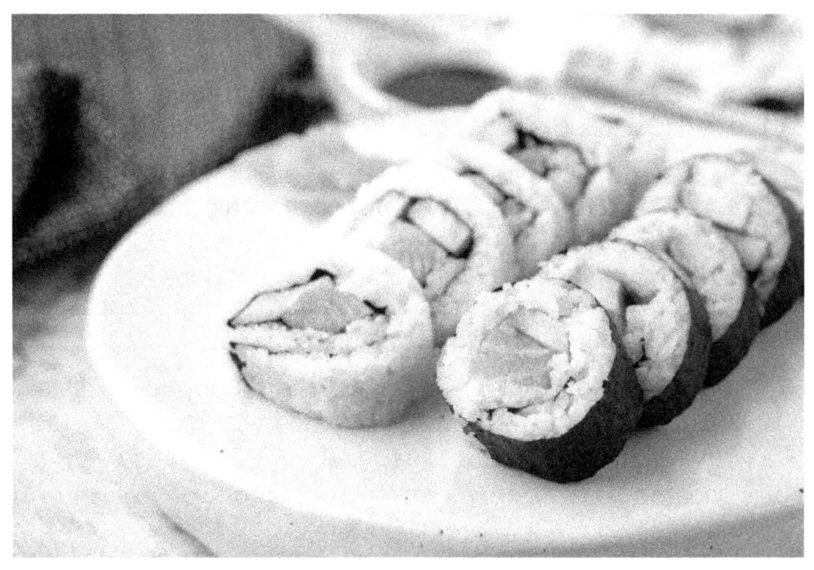

Day 20

Breakfast

Keto-friendly green smoothie with avocado and kale.

Lunch

Turkey and cheese roll-ups with mustard.

Dinner

Turkey and vegetable curry with cauliflower rice.

BREAKFAST

Keto-friendly green smoothie with avocado and kale.

INGREDIENTS

2 cups kale
2 cups almond milk
1 tablespoon lemon juice
1 avocado peeled and pitted
1 scoop protein powder I love and highly recommend this one.
1 teaspoon powdered peanut butter
½ teaspoon cinnamon powder

INSTRUCTION

Add all the ingredients to a high speed blender and puree for about 30 seconds.

Taste to adjust flavour and

serve immediately.

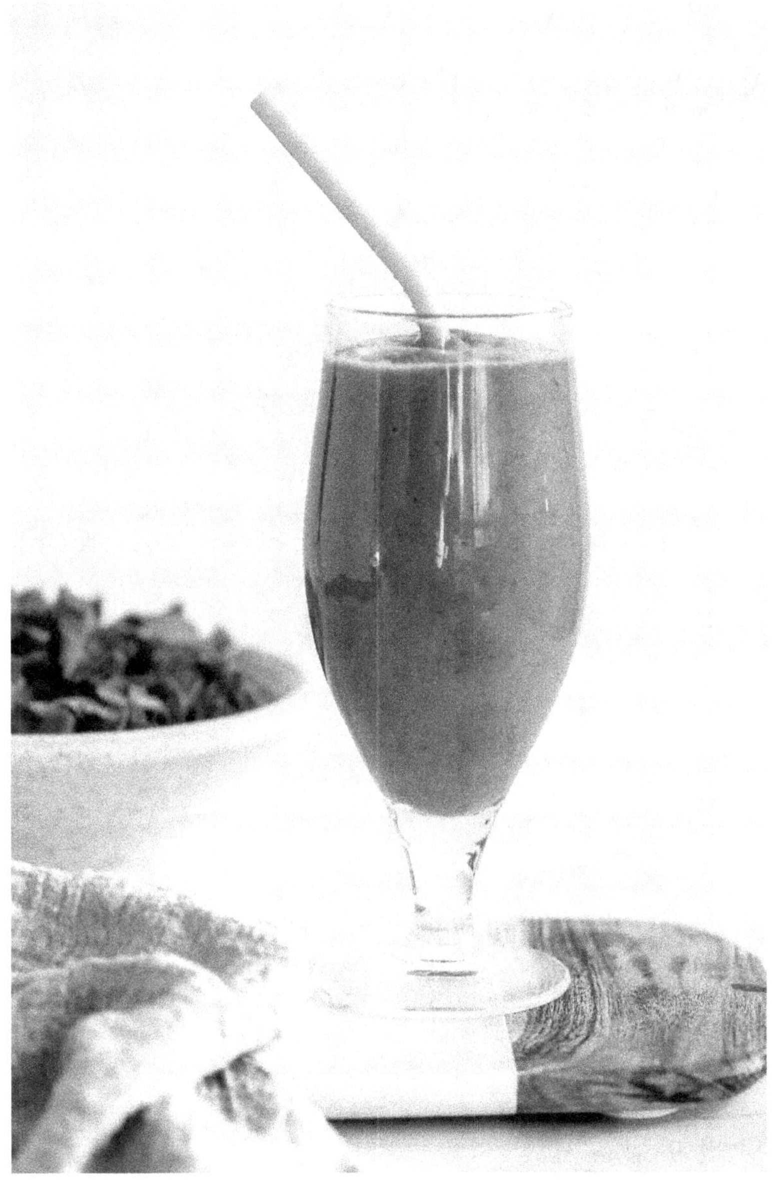

LUNCH

Turkey and cheese roll-ups with mustard.

INGREDIENTS

2-4 large flour tortillas
½ brick (8 oz) cream cheese, softened
2 tablespoons mayonaise
2 tablespoons honey mustard
¼ teaspoon salt
½ teaspoon pepper
1 large tomato, diced
1 stalk celery, diced
1 stalk green onion, thinly sliced
1 cup cheese, shredded
baby romaine lettuce or baby spinach,
⅔ pound your favorite sandwich meat, pre-sliced, more or less
to taste

INSTRUCTION

Measure your ingredients.
Add cream cheese, honey mustard, mayonnaise, salt and pepper
to a mixing bowl.
Whip until blended.
Gently fold in tomatoes, celery, green onion and shredded
cheese.
Until incorporated.
Divide and evenly spread mixture on each tortilla, almost right
to the edge. I have found large tortillas that are 8 inches up to
12 inches in size, depending on the brand. This recipe will
make 2 twelve inch tortillas. The number of tortillas you make
will also be decided depending on how much of the cream
cheese mixture you place on each tortilla.
Remove spine from romaine lettuce or spinach, if using, or
place baby romaine or baby spinach all over the entire tortilla.
I use the baby romaine or baby spinach whenever possible just
because it is easier!
Top with slices of your favorite sandwich meat to cover and
hold down the greens. You can use as many slices as you want
on each tortilla.

Roll tortillas as tightly as possible and wrap in plastic wrap or parchment paper and then tinfoil. Refrigerate for at least 4 hours, if not overnight.
When serving, unwrap and cut into ½ - ¾ inch slices.
Serve and enjoy!

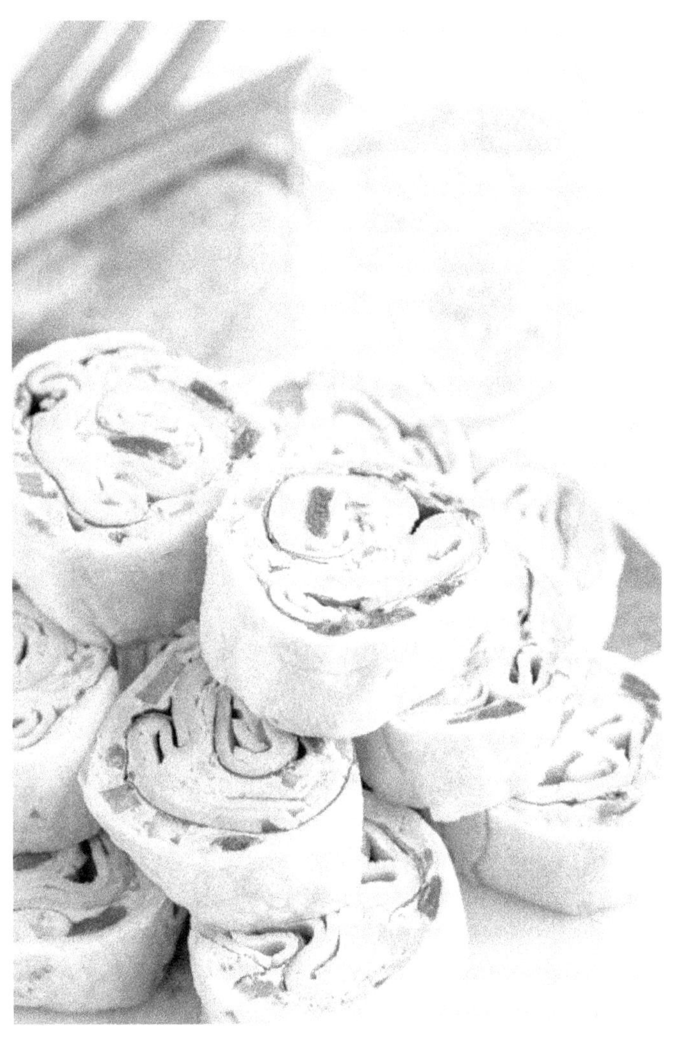

DINNER

Turkey and vegetable curry with cauliflower rice.

INGREDIENTS

half a medium-sized cauliflower

tsp of ground cumin

1 red onion, diced

2 cloves garlic, crushed

400g turkey breast (or chicken), diced into 2-3cm chunks

1 tbsp hot curry powder

1 tbsp Garam Masala

400g tin chopped tomatoes

1 cup organic chicken stock (I use Kallo)

2 green chillies, deseeded and finely sliced

3 tbsp Rapeseed oil (I use Calvia)

200g steamed broccoli

1 few handfuls spinach

fresh coriander (optional)

INSTRUCTION

To make the curry...

Heat 2 tbsp Rapeseed oil in a large, heavy-based frying pan. Add the diced red onion and cook for 3 minutes, until it softens and begins to turn translucent. Add the garlic and chillies and continue to cook for a further 2-3 minutes.
Add the spices and stir well for 2 minutes, until the fragrance is released. Add the diced turkey breast and stir well to coat well in the spices, cooking for 5 minutes or so over a medium-high heat so the meat browns.
Add the tin of chopped tomatoes and the chicken stock, cover and simmer for 25 minutes over a low heat. Check occasionally and stir as needed.
Once the timer is up and the sauce has thickened, add the cooked broccoli and spinach and cook for a further 5 minutes until hot. Serve with the 'cauli-rice' below.
To make the cauliflower rice...

Preheat the oven to 200C and get out a large, flat roasting tray. Remove the outer leaves from the cauliflower and most of the thick core. Roughly chop into large chunks.

Add a few pieces of the cauliflower chunks to the food processor at a time (as not to overload). Using the pulse setting, blitz for 30 seconds or so, until the cauliflower resembles fine rice, or couscous.

Toss the 'rice' in a drizzle of Rapeseed oil and season with a tsp of ground cumin and some freshly ground blackpepper.

Tip: don't add salt, apparently that tampers with the texture!

Spread the 'cauli-rice' out to a thin, even layer on the roasting tray, and roast in the oven at 200C for 12 minutes, mixing it up halfway through cooking.

If desired, top with some chopped fresh coriander and serve with the above curry recipe.

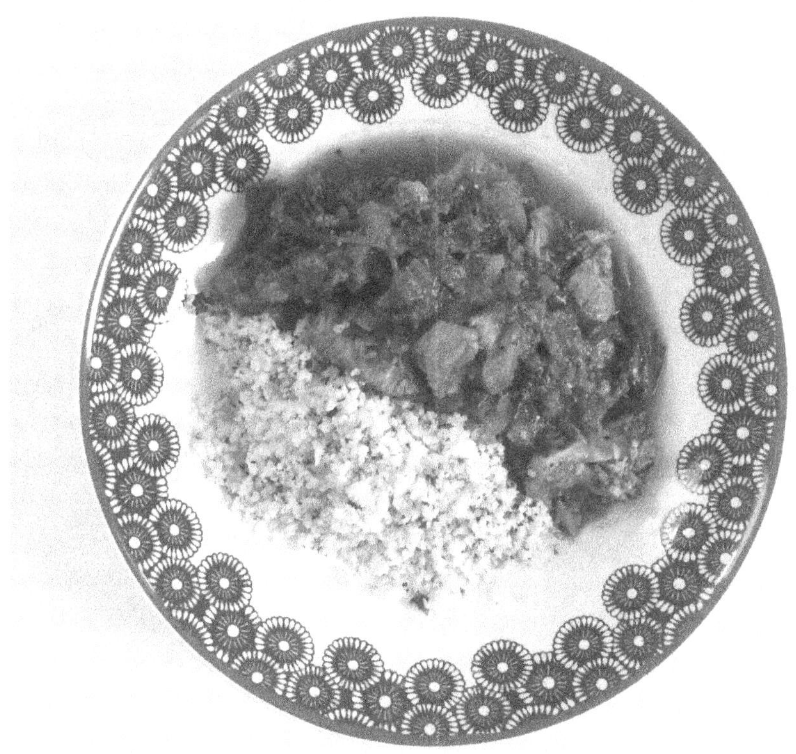

Day 21

Breakfast

Caprese omelette with tomatoes, mozzarella, and basil.

Lunch

Keto-friendly egg drop soup with vegetables.

Dinner

Lemon garlic butter chicken with green beans.

BREAKFAST

Caprese omelette with tomatoes, mozzarella, and basil.

INGREDIENTS

4 eggs (or equivalent in vegan egg substitute)
8 fresh basil leaves (or 1 tbsp dried basil)
2 cloves garlic
1/4 bell pepper
1 small- medium size tomato, diced
1/8th diced red onion
1/4 cup fresh mozzarella (or vegan cheese substitute)
salt and pepper to taste
dash oil

INSTRUCTION

Saute garlic, onion, and bell pepper in oil over medium heat for 1-2 mins in a small-medium sized frying pan, then add tomato and season with salt and pepper as desired. Cook for 4-5 minutes, until bell pepper is soft. While veggie mix is cooking, scramble 2 eggs and set aside. Cut mozzarella into slices and dice fresh basil. Once veggies are done, set aside in bowl (or whatever container is the most camping clean at the moment). Coat frying pan with more oil if needed, then pour eggs in. Tilt the pan as needed until eggs form a thin circle inside bottom of pan. Once eggs are mostly cooked, add 1/2 veggie mixture to one half of eggs. Top with mozzarella and fresh basil, fold other half of egg mixture on top to form a beautiful omelette (its ok if the egg rips, ya'll, it's still gonna taste amazing), let cheese melt, and then serve. Repeat process with the last 2 eggs and remaining veggie mix, congratulate yourself on crushing the first meal of the day, and enjoy.

Makes 2 hearty omelettes.
Use dried basil, garlic power, and onion powder if you're out of the fresh stuff. Omit the bell pepper if needed and swap fresh tomatoes for canned (if you can get your hands on a can of fire roasted tomatoes, it'll make your omelette (and your day). Throw in a dollop of ricotta cheese to add a creamy texture and serve with a side of whole-grain toast.

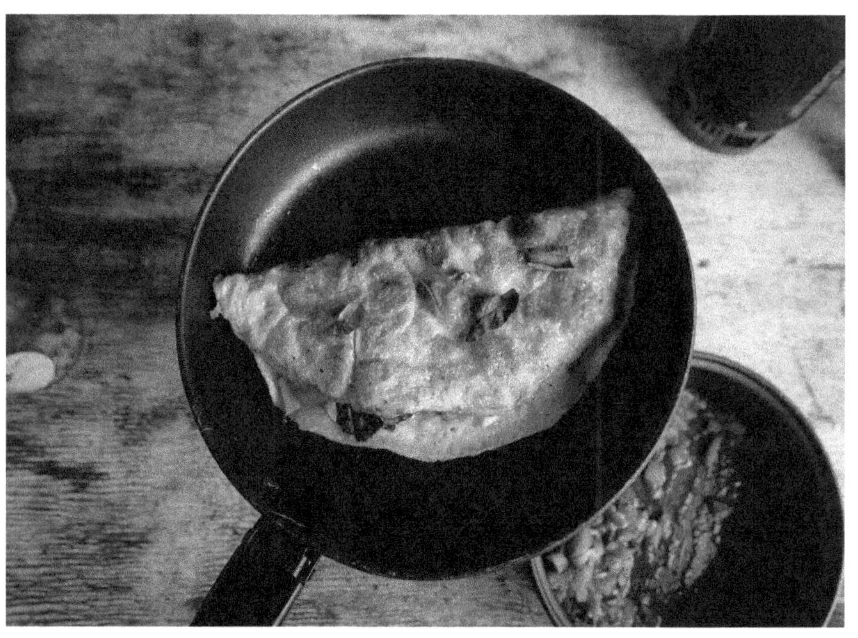

LUNCH

Keto-friendly egg drop soup with vegetables.

INGREDIENTS

4 cups Chicken broth
1 teaspoon Ginger paste
8 ounces Sliced mushrooms
1 tablespoon Soy sauce
⅓ cup Chopped green onions
3 large Eggs beaten lightly
Salt and white pepper to taste

INSTRUCTION

Add the chicken broth, ginger paste, mushrooms, soy sauce, green onions and salt and white pepper to taste in a pot over medium high heat on the stove.

Bring the mixture to a boil, and simmer for 15 minutes.

Mix the eggs in slowly, stirring as you do.

Continue to simmer a few more minutes before serving.

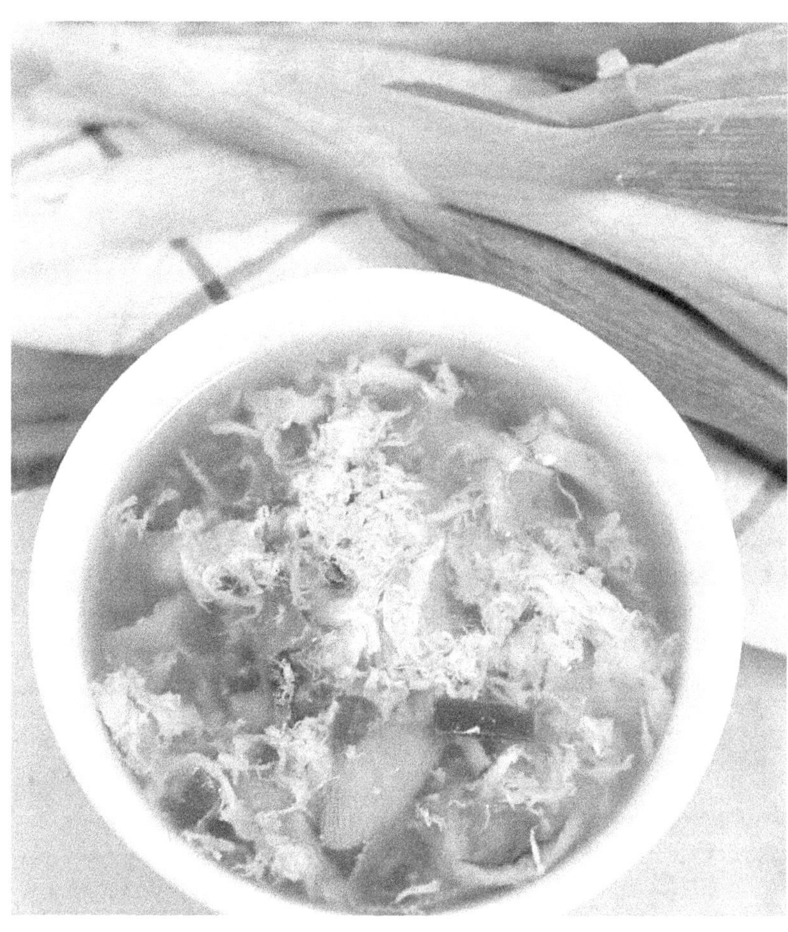

DINNER

Lemon garlic butter chicken with green beans.

INGREDIENTS

3 – 6 skinless, boneless chicken thighs
1 pound (450g) green beans, trimmed
3 tablespoons butter, divided or (ghee for paleo diet)
4 garlic cloves, minced
1 teaspoon paprika
1 teaspoon onion powder
1/4 teaspoon salt and fresh cracked black pepper
Juice of 1/2 lemon + lemon slices, for garnish
1/2 cup (125ml) chicken stock
1 tablespoon hot sauce (we used Sriracha)
1/4 teaspoon crushed red chili pepper flakes, optional
1/2 cup fresh chopped parsley

INSTRUCTION

To make the lemon garlic butter chicken thighs recipe with green beans: In a small bowl, combine onion powder, paprika, salt, and pepper. Season chicken thighs generously with the spice mixture. Set aside while you prepare green beans.

2. Arrange green beans in a microwave-safe dish with 1/2 cup (125ml) water. Cook in the microwave for 8-10 minutes, until almost done but still crisp.

3. Melt 2 tablespoons butter in a large skillet over medium-low heat. Lay the seasoned chicken thighs in one layer in the skillet. Cook for 5-6 minutes then flip and cook another 5-6 minutes, until cooked through and a cooking thermometer displays 165°F (75°C). If chicken browns too quickly, lower the heat. Adjust timing depending on the thickness. Transfer chicken to a plate and set aside.

4. In the same skillet, lower the heat and melt the remaining tablespoon of butter. Add chopped parsley, garlic, hot sauce, red crushed chili pepper flakes, and pre-cooked green beans and cook for 4 to 5 minutes, stirring regularly, until cooked to your liking. Add lemon juice and chicken stock and reduce the sauce for a couple of minutes, until slightly thickened.

5. Push green beans to the side and add cooked chicken thighs back to the pan and reheat quickly.

Adjust seasoning with pepper and serve the lemon garlic butter chicken thighs immediately, garnished with more crushed chili pepper, fresh parsley, and a slice of lemon if you like. Enjoy!

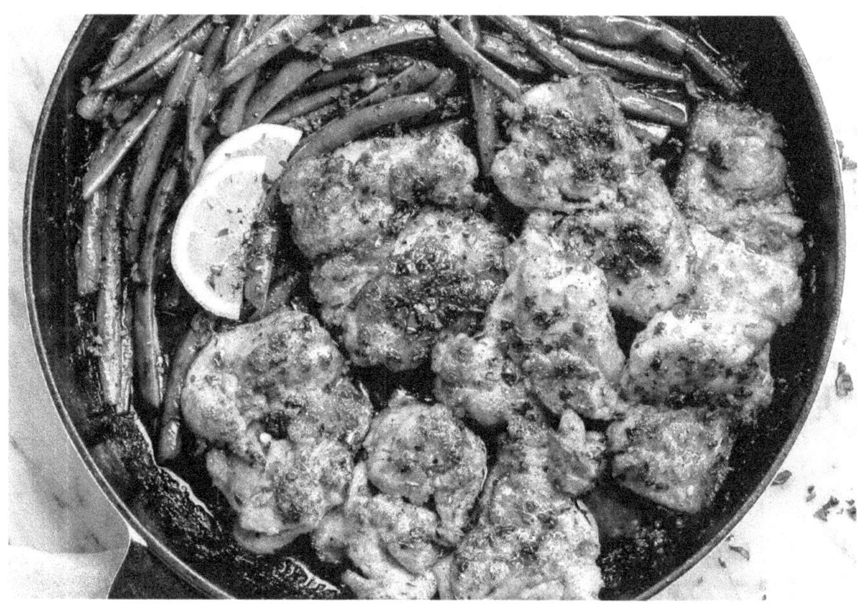

Conclusion

In the final chapters of "Complete 21 Days Weight Watcher Cookbook" by Dr. Sharon S. Lent, readers embark on a transformative culinary journey. As Lent artfully combines her expertise in health and diet, the concluding recipes not only signify the culmination of a 21-day commitment but also serve as a flavorful testament to the harmony between mindful eating and delicious indulgence. The book's conclusion beckons readers to savor not just the taste of wholesome meals but the accomplishment of a healthier lifestyle, inviting them to relish the ongoing chapters of their own wellness journey beyond the last page.

As you turn the pages towards the end of Dr. Sharon S. Lent's "Complete 21 Days Weight Watcher Cookbook," it's like reaching the summit of a culinary adventure. The final recipes not only reflect her health and diet expertise but also encapsulate the essence of a 21-day commitment to well-being. It's not just about the delicious meals; it's a celebration of making mindful choices and embracing a healthier lifestyle. So, as you savor the last bites, it's not just the taste lingering but the satisfaction of a journey well-navigated, inviting you to continue this flavorful path towards a balanced and vibrant life.

ABOUT THE AUTHOR

Dr Sharon S. Lent

Welcome to the realm of sustainable weight loss and nourishing diets! Dr. Lent, a seasoned medical professional specializing in weight loss and diet, brings a wealth of expertise to guide you on your transformative journey to a healthier you.

Meet Dr. Sharon S. Lent

With a passion for empowering individuals to achieve their health goals, Dr. Sharon S. Lent has dedicated her career to the intersection of medicine, nutrition, and well-being. Holding a Doctor of Medicine degree, her specialized focus on weight loss has allowed her to make a meaningful impact on countless lives.

Areas of Expertise

Dr. Lent is renowned for her comprehensive approach to weight management, combining medical knowledge with practical, sustainable strategies. Her expertise includes personalized diet plans, evidence-based interventions, and holistic well-being practices.

A Trusted Guide:

As a trusted guide on the journey to better health, Dr. Lent emphasizes the importance of mindful living, making choices that resonate with individual lifestyles, and fostering a positive relationship with food.

Contributions to the Field:

Beyond her clinical practice, Dr. Lent is an avid contributor to the field of weight management. Her research, articles, and contributions to reputable health publications reflect a commitment to sharing knowledge and fostering a community dedicated to wellness.

Join the Journey:

Embark on a journey towards sustainable weight loss and a nourished, balanced life with Dr. Lent. Through her insights, you'll discover practical, achievable steps that go beyond the conventional approach to dieting, paving the way for a healthier, more vibrant future.

REVIEW

Dear Reader,

We hope you're enjoying your journey with the "Complete 21-days weight watcher cookbook" Your experience matters to us, and we'd love to hear your thoughts on how the program has been for you.

Whether you've just started or are well into your transformation, your review can inspire others and help us fine-tune our approach to better suit your needs. Please take a moment to share your feedback on the "Complete 21-days weight watcher cookbook". Your insights are invaluable in shaping the success stories of our community.

Thank you for being a part of this journey with us. Your review is not just a reflection of your experience but also a beacon for others seeking a healthier lifestyle.

We appreciate your time and input.

www.ingramcontent.com/pod-product-compliance
Lightning Source LLC
Chambersburg PA
CBHW070937260726
48661CB00003B/1029